NCT
Pregnancy

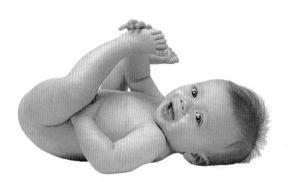

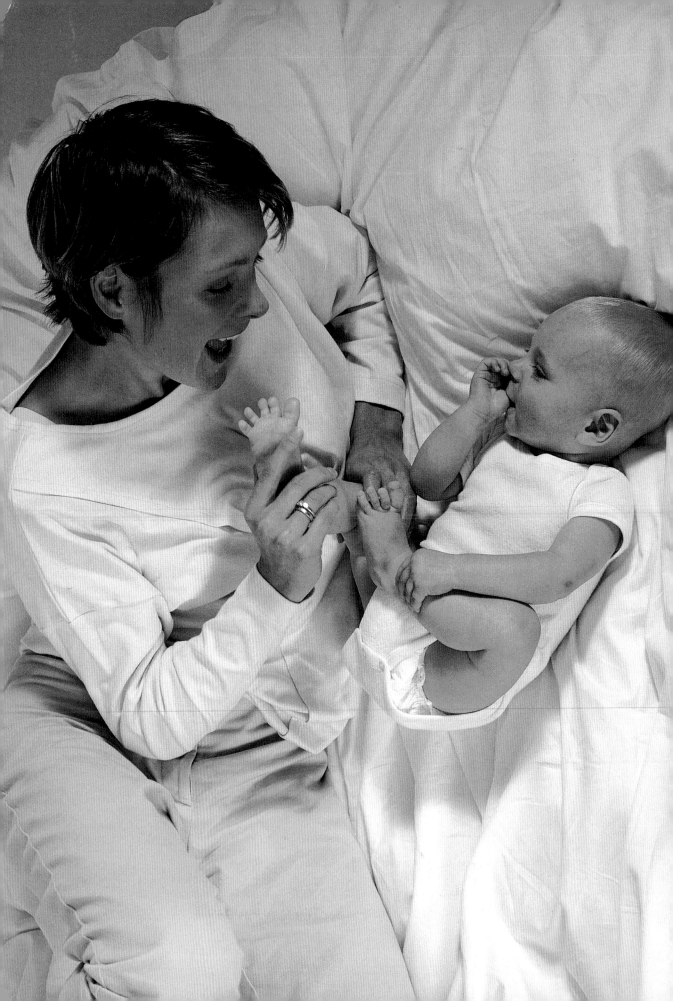

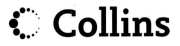

NCT Pregnancy

Edited by Daphne Metland

Photography by Anne Green-Armytage

The Essential Guide from Conception to Birth from the

NATIONAL CHILDBIRTH TRUST

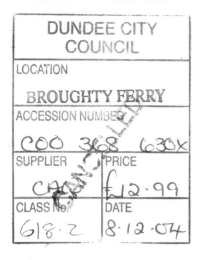
The National Childbirth Trust (NCT) offers information and support in pregnancy, childbirth and early parenthood. We aim to give every parent the chance to make informed choices. We try to make sure that our services, activities and membership are fully accessible to everyone. Donations to support our work are welcome.

National Childbirth Trust, Alexandra House, Oldham Terrace, London W3 6NH Tel: 020 8992 8637

ACKNOWLEDGEMENTS

With grateful thanks to all the beautiful women who kindly agreed to be photographed for this book! Thanks also to Formes, Blooming Marvellous, JoJo Maman Bébé, Freemans and Shaker for providing clothes and props, and to Gina Ulgen and Nicky Ralph for styling and make up.

We would also like to thank Miss Jennison, Dr Morag Martindale, Helen du Père, Jane Fleming and Cynthia Masters-Waage for their help with reading the manuscript.

PICTURE ACKNOWLEDGEMENTS

Original photography by Anne Green-Armytage
© 2000 NCT Publishing
Additional photography by Eddie Lawrence pages 28, 31, 32, 49, 84, 87, 88, 89, 92, 95, 96, 97, 99, 101, 102, 103, 104, 105, 106, 107, 111, 115
Lynn Walford pages 17, 39, 44, 45, 47, 91
George Williams pages 16, 17, 40, 58, 78, 79
Michael Bassett pages 1, 2, 68, 116
Daniel Ward pages 11, 19, 23
Chris Lane pages 9, 55

Published by Collins, an imprint of
HarperCollins*Publishers* Ltd
77–85 Fulham Palace Road, Hammersmith,
London W6 8JB
in collaboration with National Childbirth Trust
Publishing, 25–27 High Street, Chesterton,
Cambridge CB4 1ND, UK

© 2000 NCT Publishing HB
© 2004 NCT Publishing PB

A CIP catalogue record for this book is available from the British Library.

ISBN 0 00 718308 9

Design by Tim McPhee
Editorial by Sonia Leach
Project Co-ordination by Debbie Wayment and Franca Holden

Production in association with Book Production Consultants plc, 25-27 High Street, Chesterton, Cambridge, CB4 1ND, UK

Printed and bound in Italy

THE AUTHORS

DAPHNE METLAND has prepared hundreds of couples for the birth of their babies through her 15 years' work as an antenatal teacher with the National Childbirth Trust. A consumer journalist by profession, she is a regular contributor to magazines, TV and radio. After taking a break to have two children, Daphne returned to full-time journalism as editor of *Parents* magazine and is now a full-time freelance publishing consultant.

SUE ALLEN-MILLS is variously a mother, a writer and editor, and an NCT antenatal teacher, depending on what time of day it is. Before children, she was an editor of social science books. Since becoming a mother, she has worked as a writer and has been an NCT teacher since 1991. She continues to find great reward in supporting women and their partners through pregnancy and helping them to prepare for the birth of their babies.

HANNAH HULME HUNTER is a practising midwife and NCT breastfeeding counsellor. She has worked as an editor for MIDIRS (Midwives Information and Resource Service) and the NCT. She has written many articles for midwifery and parenting publications, and is the author of the *NCT Book of Safe Foods* (with Rosemary Dodds).

MARY NOLAN is a long-time NCT antenatal teacher and writer on childbirth issues, and has extended her work into schools where she explores the impact of having a baby with tomorrow's parents. In addition to writing for the midwifery journals and the popular press, Mary has worked with student nurses and midwives to highlight the needs of women during pregnancy, in labour and after the birth of their babies. Mary has recently acquired a doctorate researching approaches to preparing people for birth and early parenthood.

GILLIAN FLETCHER is author of the NCT's *Get Into Shape After Childbirth*. She's also co-author of a chapter on 'empowerment' in a recently published book for midwives and feels that this title sums up much of her antenatal teaching work – helping others to feel empowered and confident in their own abilities. As well as continuing her 26 years of NCT antenatal teaching, she now works as a freelance trainer.

ANNE GREEN-ARMYTAGE worked as a computer consultant in the City of London before rediscovering her childhood love of photography after the birth of her first child. She now works as a freelance photographer part-time, concentrating on babies, plants and gardens, not necessarily in that order, for various magazines and books. A keen supporter of the NCT, Anne has been a newsletter editor, antenatal bookings clerk and chair of her local branch.

PUBLISHER'S NOTE

In the interests of equality, we have referred to 'your baby' before and after birth throughout the text as sometimes 'he' and sometimes 'she'. We would like to thank all the couples who generously shared the story of their babies' births with us, so that we could reproduce those stories here.

We have endeavoured where possible to reproduce quotations verbatim, but where editing has been applied, the integrity of the quotation has been maintained.

EDITOR'S INTRODUCTION

Having a baby is one of the most exciting and intimidating things we ever do. It changes our body, our life and the way we view the world, for ever. Babies, especially our own babies, are so wonderful that we go on having them, despite the fears and worries about the process of pregnancy and birth.

Finding out all you can about having a baby is a really useful way of dealing with those fears and worries. Joining a National Childbirth Trust antenatal class was one of the best things I have ever done. I got so hooked on the information, the friendship and the support, that I trained as a teacher and over 15 years later I'm still teaching! My kids have grown up with pregnant couples arriving at the house each week, with dads ringing breathless and excited to tell me about the birth, and groups coming back for reunions to show off their new babies.

This book, with its lovely photographs, in-depth information and real life accounts, will guide you through your pregnancy and the early days of parenthood. It has been written so that you can dip into it for specific facts and information, settle down and read it from cover to cover, or read each section as you reach that stage of pregnancy.

I hope you find it useful and enjoy the process of becoming a parent. Always remember that – as far as your baby is concerned – you are the perfect parent!

Daphne Metland

Daphne Metland

Editor

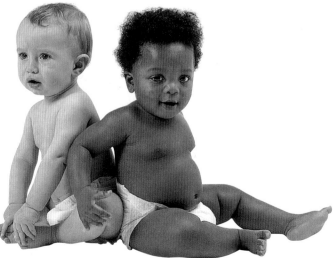

CONTENTS

First trimester   10

Conception *12*

Eating well *16*

Eating safely *18*

Staying fit *22*

Choosing antenatal care *24*

Your booking visit *26*

Talking to professionals *28*

Antenatal tests *30*

Antenatal exercises *34*

Pregnancy sickness *38*

Early pregnancy discomforts *40*

Second trimester   42

Weight gain *46*

Waterbirth *48*

Making a birth plan *50*

Labour partners *52*

Your rights at work *54*

Baby equipment *57*

Later discomforts *59*

Twins and more *62*

Pregnancy problems *64*

Your changing relationships *68*

Third trimester   70

Skills for labour *74*

What to pack for labour *78*

Going overdue *80*

Your labour and birth   82

Early first-stage labour *86*

Late first-stage labour *88*

Pain relief: helping yourself *90*

Pain relief: extra help *92*

Induction/acceleration *94*

Monitoring labour *96*

Long labours *98*

Problematic labours *100*

Second stage of labour *102*

Assisted deliveries *106*

Caesarean birth *108*

Third stage of labour *110*

You and your new baby   112

Your body after the birth *116*

Your feelings after birth *120*

Postnatal exercises *122*

The early days at home *124*

Breast or bottle? *128*

Breastfeeding *132*

Bottle-feeding *138*

Special circumstances *142*

BIRTH STORIES   148

A waterbirth at home *148*

A second home birth *150*

A big boy born in hospital *152*

An emergency caesarean *154*

Two caesarean births *156*

Vaginal birth after caesarean *158*

A birth induced in hospital *160*

Giving birth to twins *162*

A little sister born at home *164*

PREGNANCY: AN A-Z   166

RESOURCES   186

INDEX   189

FIRST TRIMESTER
0–12 WEEKS

You've done it! You've conceived a baby. The journey has begun and now you're probably feeling a whole mixture of emotions – excitement, fear, contentment, anxiety, pride or perhaps just 'so what?'

During the next 40 weeks, your body is going to go through the most extraordinary changes as your baby grows inside you.

Nine months probably seems a very long way away. This is good, because it gives you a generous amount of time to get adjusted to the idea of becoming a mother.

It's in these first few weeks that the baby's body and all its organs are formed. Growth is miraculous and speedy. The brain, spinal cord, vital organs and circulation develop now in a matter of a few weeks (see page 12). No wonder you're feeling tired! From single fertilised cell to fully formed fetus takes less than 12 weeks, and after that your baby just needs to grow and mature in the incubator of your body.

You'll need to start taking folic acid tablets (see pages 17 and 173). Don't wait until your pregnancy has been confirmed to do this. Stop smoking (see page 21). If you really can't stop,

at least cut down. The same goes for drinking: cut right down on alcohol. Many women prefer to stop completely, to be on the safe side, at least for the first 12 weeks.

It's also a good idea to avoid over-the-counter medications, both conventional and alternative treatments. If you are having any kind of medical treatment, tell your doctor or therapist that you are expecting a baby.

SAFETY

If you practise any strenuous sports, consult with your coach about the advisability of cutting down or stopping for a while. Tiredness will definitely be a factor now and you may prefer to take things easy for the first 12 weeks.

Think about whether there are any safety-at-work issues for you. See page 54 for some useful information about maternity rights at work and page 186 for more sources of help.

Relax, breathe deeply, go outside and feel yourself part of nature. Know that everything will be all right.

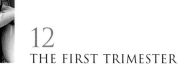

CONCEPTION

Some women seem to get pregnant almost without effort. For others, it may be the end of a long and frustrating struggle. However it happens, it can be hard at first to believe it!

It takes just one sperm to fertilise the ovum. Fertilisation may take place an hour after intercourse – or several days later. (Healthy sperm can live for 3–4 days within your body.) This single event is the start of nine months of miraculous happenings – and a lifetime of opportunities.

Following fertilisation, the ovum continues its journey down your fallopian tube to the uterus. Hormones produced by the 'corpus luteum' (which is the yellow scar left behind when the ovum was released from your ovary) prepare your body for pregnancy. Meanwhile, the cells within the ovum are beginning to divide and multiply, and the tiny sphere becomes known as a 'blastocyst'. Once in your uterus, the blastocyst burrows into the lining that has been building up since the end of your last period. The following sequence of events occurs:

• Some women bleed a little as the blastocyst embeds in the uterine lining.

• Tiny finger-like projections start to sprout from the blastocyst. Some of these will develop into the placenta (or afterbirth). The blastocyst begins to secrete a hormone called human chorionic gonadotrophin (HCG). HCG stimulates the corpus luteum to continue producing progesterone. In fact, it's the levels of HCG in your bloodstream that make the pregnancy test positive.

• Meanwhile, the cells inside the blastocyst have arranged themselves into two main groups: an outer ring of cells that form a kind of bag (known as the 'gestational sac'), and an inner group (the 'embryo'). The outer ring will eventually form the membranes that enclose the amniotic fluid in which your baby floats.

The embryo will become your baby. Tiny blood vessels are already beginning to form – and only two weeks have passed since conception (four weeks since your last monthly period or LMP).

• Your period does not start – although you may experience some mild cramps.

• Your breasts may feel tingly and full.

• Some women experience a sudden dislike of things like coffee or alcohol. Others are aware of an odd metallic taste in their mouth. Some women start to feel sick.

Further amazing changes now take place. The tiny blood vessels within the embryo connect with vessels in the primitive placenta, and blood starts to circulate. Four short weeks after conception (six weeks after your LMP), the embryo is no bigger than a grain of rice, yet head and body can be seen. Leg and arm buds appear soon afterwards.

Five weeks after conception (seven weeks since your LMP) the heart starts to beat.

• Most women are now feeling sick, as HCG levels continue to rise. (They start to fall at about 12 weeks.)

• You may feel very tired. This is probably a reaction to rising levels of progesterone.

• You may also find that you need to make visits to the toilet more often. This is because

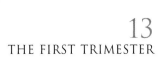

your uterus is pressing against your bladder.

A few women continue to bleed at regular monthly intervals for two to three months (occasionally even longer). This is called 'decidual bleeding', since it is bleeding from the decidua (lining of the pregnant uterus) that is not yet in contact with the embryo. By 12 weeks this bleeding generally stops.

Six weeks after conception (eight weeks after your LMP), the gestational sac containing the embryo is the size of a grape. The embryo has eyes and ears, and hands. She is moving, and the basics of all the major body systems are in place.

PREGNANCY TESTS

Some women sense they are pregnant almost before they miss a period. If this is you, trust your body and save your money.

Many women, however, prefer to know for sure whether or not they are pregnant. Most home pregnancy tests can give this assurance from as early as the first day of your missed period – just two weeks after conception.

Home pregnancy tests (available from most chemists) work by detecting the hormone HCG in urine. If HCG is present, the indicator stick will change colour, or a coloured line will appear. This means you are pregnant.

A negative result – no colour change – may mean that you are not pregnant. Or it may mean that there is not yet enough HCG in your urine to give a positive result. It might be a good idea to wait a few days and then, if your period has still not started, try another test.

Home pregnancy tests are expensive – about £10 for two tests. Free pregnancy tests may be available in GP's surgeries, family planning clinics, and antenatal clinics, but these tests are generally not as sensitive as a home test. You may not get a positive result until two weeks after your period should have started.

TRYING FOR A BABY?

Check your weight. It's harder to get pregnant if you're overweight or underweight.

Try to eat properly. See page 16. Take a folic acid supplement, but eat foods rich in folic acid too. See page 17.

Stop smoking, or cut right down. Protecting your baby from smoke is probably the single most beneficial thing you can do for her.

Cut alcohol right down. Find more information on page 20.

Don't take any drugs, over-the-counter or otherwise, while you're trying to conceive, although paracetamol is considered safe.

Ask your GP for a blood test to make sure you're immune to German measles.

Guard against certain infections:

- Toxoplasmosis and listeriosis are described on page 18.
- Chlamydia psittaci is a disease of sheep. If you suspect you might be pregnant, don't have any contact with lambing ewes, newborn lambs or even clothes worn during lambing.

Women with high blood pressure, diabetes or epilepsy may need to see their specialist, since pregnancy can make these conditions worse.

Work conditions that may not be suitable include heavy lifting, operating vibrating machinery, standing for long periods, and exposure to excessive heat, cold or noise. Toxic substances that should be avoided include solvents, pesticides, herbicides, lead, anaesthetic gases, radiation, biological hazards, and pharmaceuticals.

If you are pregnant, reading this panel may make you feel anxious. Try not to worry! Your body is designed for pregnancy and babies are generally very resilient.

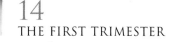

The weeks of pregnancy are always counted from the first day of your last menstrual period (LMP). In other words, the counting starts from two weeks *before* you conceive. This method has become standard practice because relatively few women can pinpoint the day of conception – but most can recall their last period.

Human pregnancy (or gestation) lasts, on *average*, 40 weeks from the LMP.

The LMP method works well if you have a regular menstrual cycle. But some women have irregular periods, or are confused by bleeding in early pregnancy. The LMP method may not be helpful in these circumstances, so an ultrasound scan to estimate gestation may be offered.

Other women may have regular periods but may, in the month they conceive, ovulate much later (or earlier) than normal. This may explain why the due date suggested following a scan might sometimes disagree with your due date according to your LMP.

Scan technicians estimate the length of pregnancy by measuring the embryo, and comparing these results with a chart of standard sizes/gestations. The earlier the scan is performed, the more accurate these comparisons. Even so, scan 'dates' are only accurate to within five days. A scan later than 20–24 weeks cannot accurately assess gestation.

Remember – even if you do not know your LMP and your due date is estimated by scan, the weeks of your pregnancy will still be counted from two weeks before conception.

ESTIMATED DATE OF DELIVERY (EDD)

Midwives like to calculate the due date by adding 9 months and 7 days to the LMP. But please note that the date you will be given is an *estimated* date. Your baby may be born any time between 37 and 42 weeks and still be considered 'due' by most people.

MIXED FEELINGS

Many women are shocked by the mixed emotions they experience when they realise they are pregnant. Usually there is delight and amazement – but so often this joy is clouded by anxiety, panic and even depression. You may wonder if you've done the right thing.

In the short term, these feelings are very normal. After all, becoming pregnant is probably the single most life-changing event of our lives. Furthermore, the start of pregnancy is a time of enormous hormonal upheaval – and it takes time for your body to adjust to this.

You are not abnormal – and you are not alone. Find somebody to talk to – a friend who has experienced pregnancy herself, an older woman, or your partner. And remember that midwives are there for women, whatever their stage of pregnancy.

BLEEDING IN EARLY PREGNANCY

Bleeding does not necessarily mean that you are going to miscarry. In fact, only one in every ten women who bleeds in early pregnancy will go on to lose her baby.

However, do call your GP or midwife if:
• You lose more than a few spots of bright red blood.
• You lose a large amount of blood of whatever colour.
• You have abdominal (low tummy) pain or severe backache.
• You have pain passing urine, or an unusual vaginal discharge.
• You are very anxious about what may be happening.

Most women prefer to rest in bed, or on a sofa, if they are bleeding – although there is no research evidence that doing so will prevent a miscarriage happening. Using pads rather than tampons will make it easier to assess blood loss and reduce the risk of infection. (There's more information on bleeding in the later stages of pregnancy on page 66.)

IF THINGS GO WRONG

Sadly, nearly one in every five confirmed pregnancies will miscarry in the first 12 weeks of pregnancy.

There are many possible causes of an early miscarriage:

• Chromosome problems – the embryo fails to develop normally.

• Implantation problems – the blastocyst is unable to embed securely in the uterus, or the placenta fails to develop.

• Endocrine problems – the hormones needed to sustain the pregnancy are inadequate.

• Maternal illness – rubella, toxoplasmosis, influenza, uncontrolled diabetes, and so on.

• Environmental factors – smoking, some drugs, excessive alcohol, x-rays.

• Abnormal immune response – the mother's body 'rejects' the embryo.

If you miscarry, try not to blame yourself or others. A miscarriage is rarely anybody's fault. There is no evidence that miscarriages are caused by not resting enough, having sex, or a past termination. There is a 90% chance that your next pregnancy will be fine.

Physical recovery after an early miscarriage is usually quick, although doctors recommend that you wait until you have had at least one normal period before trying again.

However, emotional recovery may take much longer. Feelings of loss, helplessness and guilt are normal, and many women find they need time to acknowledge and mourn the lost pregnancy, before moving on once more.

See page 64 for more information and discussion about losing a baby.

ACTION PLAN

See your doctor to arrange your antenatal care and get your pregnancy confirmed. In some areas you'll see a midwife. Ask her if you want to know about any special tests or need help with symptoms such as pregnancy sickness.

Ask for form FW8 for free prescriptions.

Arrange for any special tests you would like to have (see page 30).

Make an appointment to see the dentist. Treatment is free now and until your baby is a year old.

Planning a holiday? Check vaccinations. Most cannot be given during pregnancy and remember that some exotic holiday destinations may not be a good idea because of the risk of malaria.

You may want to tell your employers that you're pregnant, so that they can alter your hours if necessary or let you have time off for appointments. On the other hand, you may want to keep the news to yourself until you're past the three-month mark.

9–12 WEEKS

Attend your first antenatal appointment (see page 26). You'll meet a midwife and have a chance to ask questions and get information. See page 28 for help with this.

Book your NCT antenatal classes, they can get very busy – see page 42.

If there's any doubt about dates, you may be offered an ultrasound scan.

Some tests, such as an early ultrasound scan to screen for some abnormalities, may be carried out now (see page 30).

Start some exercises (see page 34) and try to spend some time every day relaxing completely and focusing on your baby.

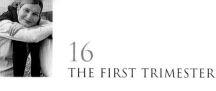

EATING WELL

Eating a full and balanced diet is one of the most vital contributions you can make to the health of your baby. It is second only to protecting her from the effects of smoking.

Enjoying your food is more than just taking in nutrients – good food shared with others is one of life's pleasures. But now you are sharing every mouthful with your baby.

Healthy eating matters because eating well before, during and after pregnancy provides for your baby as she develops and grows, maintains your health during pregnancy, builds up stores of nutrients for use when needed, prepares your body for breastfeeding, boosts your immunity to illness and infection, protects you and your baby from some of the effects of environmental pollution and establishes a healthy pattern for family eating in the years to come!

FRUIT AND VEGETABLES

You can't eat too much of this food group. Bursting with vitamins and minerals, fruit and vegetables are also an important source of 'antioxidants' – nutrients that help protect our bodies from cancer, heart disease and the effects of pollution. They're good for fibre, too.

Don't worry if you can't always buy fresh – frozen, canned and dried fruit and vegetables are virtually as good. Keep a bag of mixed frozen vegetables in the freezer to add to soup. Top breakfast cereals with tinned raspberries or dried, no-soak apricots. Use fruit that is past its peak in 'smoothies' – well chilled, low-fat bio yoghurt whisked with mashed fruit.

Eat at least five portions* of fruit and vegetables each day. Add an extra portion whilst you're breastfeeding.

*1 piece of fruit (apple, orange and so on); a heaped bowl of salad; 2–3 tablespoons of vegetables; a handful of dried fruit; small glass of fruit juice.

STARCHY CARBOHYDRATES

Not to be confused with sugary carbohydrates, starchy carbohydrates provide long-term energy and vitality – plus vitamins, minerals, protein and fibre. Sugary carbohydrates (cakes, biscuits, confectionery and

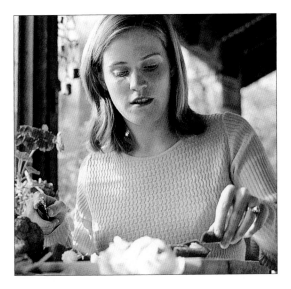

sweet desserts) give only short-term energy and little else of value.

Aim for an average of six servings* of starchy carbohydrates throughout the day. Eat to appetite: your energy needs increase late in pregnancy and while breastfeeding.

*2 slices of bread; a bowl of breakfast cereal; 6 tablespoons of cooked pasta; 4 tablespoons of rice; 2 fist-sized potatoes or yam.

PROTEIN

Growing your baby during pregnancy increases your need for protein, which can be animal or vegetable in origin.

Vegetable protein foods are low in saturated fats and high in fibre – but a less concentrated source of protein. You therefore need to eat bigger portions and a wider variety.

You need 2–3 servings* of animal protein a day, or three servings of vegetable protein.

*2 slices of meat or poultry; 1 small lamb or pork chop; ½–1 fillet of fish; 2 eggs; 3 tablespoons of cooked beans or chick peas; one-third of a 420g tin of baked beans; 100g hummus; one-third of a packet of Tofu.

DAIRY PRODUCE

Aim for three servings* of dairy produce each day. Add an extra portion while breastfeeding.

*200ml of milk; a small yoghurt; half a small tub of cottage cheese; a 2oz piece of hard cheese.

If you don't eat dairy foods, then non-milk foods rich in calcium include: tinned fish, soya milk, spinach, spring greens, chick peas, kidney beans and baked beans.

Iron is important for helping your red blood cells transport oxygen, so get your iron naturally with iron-rich foods.*
*lean meat; eggs; dark poultry; iron-fortified breakfast cereals; sardines; cashew nuts; wholemeal bread; lentils; chick peas; baked beans; leafy green vegetables; sunflower seeds; dried fruit; baked potatoes.

Make the most of the iron in your diet by:
• Combining iron-rich foods with vitamin C foods (meat and vegetables, baked beans and sliced tomato, breakfast cereals and fruit).
• Drinking tea and coffee at least half an hour before a meal – or two hours afterwards. If you have these drinks too close to a meal they tend to block your iron uptake.

Folic acid: as well as taking folic acid tablets, try to eat more foods rich in folic acid.*
*fortified breakfast cereals, bread and other fortified foods (look for the 'F'); green leafy vegetables (don't overcook); peas, beans and cauliflower; citrus and kiwi fruit.

Vitamin D: ask your GP about taking a supplement of vitamin D if you don't drink milk, or eat milk-based foods, oily fish or eggs; you rarely go out of doors between 11am and 3pm; you always cover your arms, legs and head when outside; you live in the north.

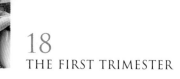

EATING SAFELY

Nowadays there seem to be so many rules surrounding what you can and can't do during pregnancy. Understanding why will help you decide what to do for yourself.

The placenta is an amazing organ. It sustains, nurtures and protects your baby throughout pregnancy, but it has its limitations. Viruses (for example, rubella and chickenpox), and some bacteria (such as listeria) and some parasites (like Toxoplasma gondii) are able to pass through it.

Your immune system also changes subtly during pregnancy. Your body has to keep a balance between acceptance of your pregnancy (remember that your baby is genetically half 'foreign' to you) and protection against illness and infection. Sometimes the balance is such that a pregnant woman may become ill when a non-pregnant woman may be fine.

There are a number of infections that you will need to guard against because they can be passed on to your unborn baby.

Toxoplasmosis is an infection you can catch from eating undercooked meat or handling cat faeces. Listeria can be caught through eating unpasteurised soft cheese or unwashed fruit and salmonella causes food poisoning.

All this may seem very alarming – and pregnant women do need to be careful – but remember human beings are already immune to numerous illnesses and infections and, more often than not, this immunity remains strong during pregnancy and is passed to the baby. Although the effects of toxoplasmosis and listeria can be tragic, both are relatively rare complications of pregnancy.

GUARDING AGAINST LISTERIA

Follow the rules of safe food handling (see box)
• Re-heat convenience foods very carefully, following the manufacturer's instructions.
• Avoid soft, ripened cheeses, blue-veined cheeses, feta cheese, all unpasteurised cheeses, and fresh paté.
• Avoid pies, pastries, poultry, and other cold buffet/picnic foods sold loose.
• Wash all salad ingredients carefully.
• Avoid ready-made salads and coleslaw at buffet meals and deli counters.
  But these foods are considered safe:
• Hard cheeses (Cheddar and so on) and processed cheeses (Dairylea, Philadelphia).
• Cottage cheese, crème fraiche, commercially sold yoghurt and cream.
• Tinned paté, meat paste in jars, any pasteurised paté (but not liver paté).
• Cold pies, pasties and salads that are packaged, date-stamped and bought from a reputable shop.

SAFE FOOD HANDLING

• Keep germs out of food – clean food, clean hands, clean kitchen.
• Stop germs multiplying in food – cool quickly, store chilled.
• Destroy any germs in food – cook or re-heat thoroughly.
• Eat food as soon as possible once prepared.

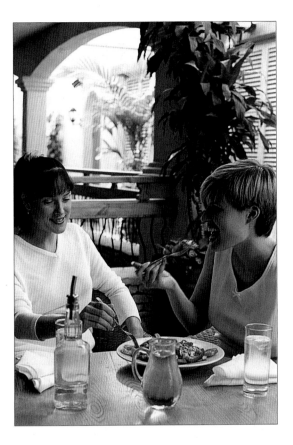

AVOIDING TOXOPLASMOSIS

Follow the rules of safe food handling (see box)
• Wash raw vegetables and store away from other foods.
• Cook meat and poultry thoroughly (there should be no pink meat, and the juices should run clear).
• Avoid raw meats such as salami and pastrami.
• Wear gloves for gardening.
• Wear gloves to handle cat litter (better still, get somebody else to do this job).
• Ask your GP early in pregnancy for a blood test to check your immunity to toxoplasmosis.

If you think you have come in contact with toxoplasmosis or listeria, contact your GP or hospital doctor urgently. Infection can be confirmed with a blood test, and drug treatment may limit the harm to your baby.

SALMONELLA FOOD POISONING

Follow the rules of safe food handling (see box)
• Avoid foods made with raw or undercooked eggs – meringue, sorbet, mousse, cake mix, home-made mayonnaise (although commercially produced pasteurised mayonnaise in a sealed jar is quite safe).
• Cook eggs until yolk and white are firm.
• Avoid soft, whipped ice cream sold from vans and kiosks.
• Avoid raw or undercooked shellfish (a potent source of food poisoning at the best of times!).
• Avoid unpasteurised milk from cows, sheep or goats (untreated milk may contain listeria and other bacteria, as well as salmonella).

THE VITAMIN A PROBLEM

Retinol vitamin A may harm your developing baby.

Avoid eating liver, and foods made with liver such as paté. These may contain dangerously high levels of retinol vitamin A. Avoid vitamins or fish oil supplements that contain the 'retinol' form of vitamin A.

THE PEANUT QUESTION

For reasons we don't fully understand, a few people suffer severe allergic reactions if they eat even tiny quantities of peanut.

Experts think that this allergy may develop during pregnancy or (less likely) breastfeeding. They feel that the incidence of peanut allergy may be reduced if certain women avoid eating peanuts and peanut products at these times. This does not apply to all mothers. You do not have to avoid peanuts unless you or your partner, or any existing children, suffer from asthma, eczema, hayfever, or other allergies.

ALCOHOL – HOW MUCH?

There is now some evidence that moderate drinking (up to a limit of 10 units of alcohol per week) may harm your baby. Research shows that drinking this amount has not been proved to be completely safe.

Moreover, if you drink more than 10–15 units per week throughout the first 12 weeks of pregnancy, your baby may have abnormalities of her heart, kidneys or other organs. If you drink over this limit later in pregnancy, she may not grow well and her IQ may be reduced.

The risks associated with alcohol are increased if you also smoke or have a poor diet.

The jury is still out on exactly how much alcohol is safe: it is unlikely that your baby will have been harmed by one or two episodes of heavy drinking before you knew you were pregnant. Experts are still not sure whether or not heavy drinking may cause a miscarriage.

The National Childbirth Trust recommends that further research is needed. In the meantime it may be wise to avoid alcohol. Other doctors and midwives feel that because the picture is still so unclear, the only safe limit is no alcohol at all. Many women settle on a 'happy medium' of no alcohol during the first 12 weeks, then a limit of one or two units a week at most thereafter.

If you're used to drinking a lot of alcohol, and find it hard to stop now that you are pregnant, please do get help: talk to your midwife or GP, or phone the AA Helpline on 0845 7697555 and speak to someone non-judgmental who can give tips on cutting down.

Don't forget – a unit of alcohol will have more effect on a small woman and her baby, than on a larger woman.

TAKING CARE WITH DRUGS

'Drugs' means anything you take to prevent or relieve symptoms – whether it is swallowed, injected, massaged on to skin, breathed in – or applied in any other way to your body. This includes alternative (or complementary) remedies and treatments, as well as conventional medications.

Many women need to take drugs to control or treat a long-term illness or medical condition. If possible, discuss your medication with your GP or specialist before you get pregnant. If this has not been possible, contact your doctor urgently as soon as you suspect you are pregnant. Together you can balance the benefits and risks of your drugs, and (if necessary) find safer alternatives.

Always tell anybody treating you that you are pregnant – even if you think it is obvious.

Always ask your GP or a pharmacist for advice before buying or taking any 'over-the-counter' drugs – even things like cold remedies or headache tablets. There is no evidence that normal doses of ordinary paracetamol causes problems.

Remember that your baby is being formed during the first 12 weeks of pregnancy (later she basically just grows). Try to avoid taking any drugs during this crucial time.

UNITS OF ALCOHOL

One unit of alcohol is:

- ½ pint of ordinary strength beer, lager or cider OR
- ¼ pint of strong beer or cider OR
- 1 small glass (100ml) of wine OR
- 1 measure (25ml) of spirits OR
- 1 small sherry glass (55ml) of sherry, port or vermouth.

Aromatherapy in pregnancy

Aromatherapy is currently one of the most popular of the alternative therapies. It involves the use of concentrated essential plant oils, widely sold in chemists and health shops. It can be very effective – but it can also be dangerous.

These – and other – oils may cause harm to you or your baby: lavender, marjoram, rosemary, sage, jasmine and camomile.

If you are interested in trying aromatherapy during pregnancy, please consider getting advice from a qualified aromatherapist (see Resources, page 186).

Cannabis

Although there is no research linking cannabis use with disabilities in babies, regular use of this drug during pregnancy may cause premature birth, or cause your baby to be jumpy or irritable during the first weeks of her life. It can also mean that your baby develops more slowly than is usual in her early years.

Caffeine

Caffeine is a stimulant drug found in coffee, tea and cola. Research has linked excessive amounts of caffeine with miscarriage, birth defects and slow growth of babies during pregnancy – although the results are somewhat confused.

'Too much' caffeine means more than 4–5 cups of instant coffee OR 2–3 cups of filtered coffee OR 5–6 cups of tea a day.

Smoking

Think what smoking does to your baby:

• It stunts her growth by reducing oxygen levels and narrowing the blood vessels in the placenta – small babies are not easier to give birth to, they are often ill, weak babies.
• It makes her heart beat unhealthily fast.
• It fills the amniotic fluid in which she floats with cancer-causing chemicals.
• It increases her chance of cot death.
• It reduces her chance of a normal, healthy, lively childhood.

Is a cigarette really worth it?

How to stop

It can be done! One in every three women who smoke will give up early in pregnancy. It may not be easy – but there's a lot of support and goodwill out there to help you along.

Ask your midwife what help is available locally for smokers who want to quit.

See Resources (page 186) for useful national organisations to contact.

FOLLOW THE TEN STEPS TO QUITTING SMOKING:

1. Make a date and stick to it.
2. Keep busy to help take your mind off cigarettes.
3. Drink plenty of fluids.
4. Get more active. Exercise helps you relax and can boost your morale.
5. Think positively. Withdrawal can be unpleasant but it is a sign that your body is recovering from the effects of tobacco.
6. Change your routine. Perhaps you should avoid the break-room at work if there are lots of smokers around you.
7. No excuses. Don't use a crisis to be an excuse for just one cigarette.
8. Pamper yourself. This is important!
9. Be careful what you eat. Try not to snack on fatty foods.
10. Take one day at a time. Each day without a cigarette is good news for your health, your pocket – and your baby.
(Taken from The Quitline's *Quit Guide to Stopping Smoking*, available from The Quitline, freephone: 0800 002200, web site: http://www.healthnet.org.uk/quit/guide)

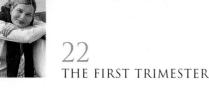

STAYING FIT

Today, most pregnant women continue to exercise and play sport, work and travel. After all – why not? If you take sensible precautions you can still enjoy your freedom.

Many women find that pregnancy is a really good time to take stock of their own health and wellbeing. Getting more exercise should be part of this. Do try to build some sort of exercise into your daily routine.

Ask your midwife if there are any antenatal exercise or yoga classes nearby, or enquire at the local leisure centre or gym. Find out if your local swimming pool has 'aquanatal' classes (exercises in water, suitable for non-swimmers as well as swimmers) – or just go swimming by yourself when the pool is quiet.

Start any exercise slowly, and build up gradually. Exercise until you feel warm and 'glowing', and are breathing a bit faster than normal. Slow down or rest for a few minutes every 15 minutes.

Know when to stop. Check your pulse regularly during exercise and slow down if it reaches 140 beats per minute.

Exercise in pregnancy relieves many of the minor ailments of pregnancy, helps improve posture and flexibility, tones and strengthens your muscles, may help prevent excessive weight gain, makes giving up smoking easier and gets you out and about.

WHY YOU NEED TO BE CAREFUL

Risks to you:
The pregnancy hormone 'relaxin' prepares your body for childbirth by softening and loosening your joints and ligaments. Soft tissue injuries such as sprains and twists are more likely than at other times and the risk of back injuries increases.

As your baby grows, your abdomen enlarges. Your centre of gravity changes, and your balance may be affected. Falls may be more likely.

Risks to your baby:
Impacts and falls may cause damage to your abdomen and, possibly, your baby.

Avoid down-hill skiing, water skiing, high diving, climbing, and all contact sports and competitive team games (netball, hockey).

If you get very hot, your baby also gets hot. Over-heating early in pregnancy may possibly affect your baby's neural (nerve) development.

Avoid saunas, steam baths and hot tubs. Stop exercising if you get very hot (rather than just warm). Drink plenty of fluids before, during and after exercise.

Sustained, vigorous exercise may affect the blood supply to your baby, by diverting blood away from the uterus to the leg muscles. If you get very breathless, the amount of oxygen in your blood is reduced. Your baby's growth may be affected.

Avoid exercising to the point of exhaustion. Stop before you are gasping for breath and your heart is pounding. Rest for a few minutes every 15 minutes.

Avoid vigorous exercise if you have had:
• Two or more miscarriages.
• Any problems in any of your previous

pregnancies with the growth of your baby.
- Any bleeding or high blood pressure in this pregnancy.
- Twins or placenta praevia diagnosed in this pregnancy.

CAR SAFETY

Pregnant women are not exempt from seat belt legislation. You must wear your seat belt throughout pregnancy. Place the lap section of the belt below your bump and tighten to fit across your hips. The diagonal section should run between your breasts. Adjust your seat backwards if the seat belt gets too short!

AIR TRAVEL

Most airlines have an upper limit beyond which they refuse to carry a pregnant woman, generally 34–36 weeks. Earlier in pregnancy (maybe 28 weeks onwards) airlines may ask you to supply a doctor's letter. These conditions vary considerably – so do please check with your travel agent or the airline.

Once in the air, the biggest risk to the pregnant traveller is that of thrombosis – the formation of a blood clot in a leg vein. Thrombosis is a rare, but very serious complication of any pregnancy. The risk of thrombosis is increased by immobility and dehydration.
- Try to book a bulkhead or aisle seat to give you some extra leg room.
- Drink plenty of (non-alcoholic) fluids before and during the flight.
- Get up and walk about for a few minutes every hour or so.
- Some obstetricians recommend taking aspirin before very long flights, to reduce the risk of clotting – but don't do this without discussing it first with your doctor.

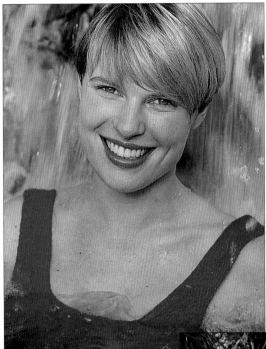

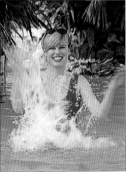

EXOTIC HOLIDAYS

Most holiday and travel insurance packages specifically exclude pregnancy, and emergency maternal and neonatal care elsewhere may be prohibitively expensive.

No vaccination should be given lightly. This is particularly true in pregnancy. Protective immunoglobulins (for example, tetanus, rabies and hepatitis A) are considered safe, but vaccines (against, for example, polio, diphtheria and meningitis) should only be given if there is no alternative.

An attack of malaria may cause late miscarriage or preterm labour. We do not know how safe anti-malaria drugs are during pregnancy.

'Traveller's diarrhoea' may be more common during pregnancy, and not all drugs normally used to treat it are considered safe in pregnancy.

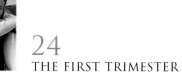

CHOOSING ANTENATAL CARE

Choosing your antenatal care is one of the earliest things you'll need to do when you become pregnant. Different areas of the country have different ranges of care available.

Antenatal care involves you being seen by a midwife or doctor at regular intervals during your pregnancy to check that all's well with you and your baby. It includes being offered a range of tests (see pp 30–33). It also gives you the opportunity of asking questions about your pregnancy and the birth of your baby and to talk about any worries or concerns you may have.

Things to think about or find out about:
• Who would you like to have for your antenatal care? A midwife, whom you can get to know, or your GP, who may already be a friend? Would you like your medical carers to be female?
• Would you like to be seen at home or would you prefer to go to hospital or to a clinic?

CHOOSING A HOSPITAL

In some areas, if you decide to have your baby in hospital, you can choose which hospital to go to.

• Talk to other women who've had babies recently about their experiences of the different hospitals.
• Find out if the hospitals have the sorts of facilities you want – for example, a 24-hour anaesthetist or a birthing pool.
• Go and look round them to see what the atmosphere is like.
• Find out what their policies are.
• How easy is it for you to get to them?

Where will you feel more comfortable? Which is easiest for you to get to during the day?
• Do you have any special healthcare needs, or any restrictions on your mobility?
• Where would you like your baby to be born? (See facing page.)
• What's available in your area?

YOUR OPTIONS

Your GP will talk to you about your options for your antenatal care when you go to see him or her to let them know that you're pregnant. Tell them if you have any particular preferences or needs. If they don't mention a type of care that you'd like, ask if it's available, or if you can go elsewhere to get it.

If your GP can't give you all the information you need, contact your local hospital, or talk to other women you know who are pregnant or have recently had babies. Your local Community Health Council (look in the phone book) and support organisations like the NCT can also help.

CHANGING YOUR MIND

If you opt for one type of care early on in your pregnancy, then find that you change your mind later on, you can always switch to another type. If you run into any problems in doing this, contact the Director of Midwifery Services at your District Health Authority.

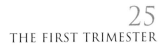

TYPES OF ANTENATAL CARE

There are several different types of care that you might be able to have when you are expecting a baby, although not all of them are available in all areas.

Type of care and its availability	Who provides it	Where it's given	Who's with you in labour
Community-based care Widely available	Your community midwife and your GP	Either at home or at your surgery or clinic	Your community midwife or hospital midwife
Shared care Widely available	Your community midwife and your GP. You have one or two appointments with a hospital doctor	As for community-based care, except you go to hospital to see the hospital doctor for one or two appointments	Your community midwife or hospital midwife
Home care (for a home birth) Available everywhere	Your community midwife. Your GP may be involved but doesn't have to be. May involve a visit to a hospital consultant	At home, or sometimes in a local clinic	Your community midwife at home
Hospital care Available everywhere, if you need it because you have medical problems or have had problems in a previous pregnancy. You can also choose to pay for private care from a hospital doctor	A hospital doctor	In a hospital clinic. In hospital (private care)	A hospital midwife and maybe a doctor
Team midwifery care Not available in all areas	A small team of community midwives. You may have one of these as 'your' midwife, but you'll also see others in the team	At home or at your surgery or clinic. In hospital or at home	Your midwife, or one of the other midwives in the team, will assist at home or in hospital
'One-to-one' midwifery care Only available in a few areas	One or two community midwives	At home or at your surgery or clinic	One of the midwives in hospital or at home
Independent care Not available in all areas. You have to pay	An independent midwife, who is professionally qualified but who works outside the NHS	At home, or possibly in a birthing centre	Your midwife at home, in a birthing centre, or in hospital

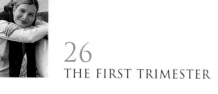

YOUR BOOKING VISIT

One of the things that your GP will arrange for you when you go to see him or her when you're first pregnant is your first meeting with your midwife or 'booking visit'.

This appointment is designed for your carers to find out about you, your general health and your pregnancy, and to see if there are any special forms of care that you need. The booking visit usually takes place when you're between 11 and 13 weeks' pregnant. You may be asked to go to a hospital clinic or to your GP's surgery, or your midwife may visit you at home. At the clinic or surgery you may be seen by a doctor as well as by a midwife.

PREPARING FOR IT

• What questions do you want to ask? Write them down as you think of them so you don't forget them.
• Arrange for someone to go with you if you think that'll make you feel more comfortable.
• You're entitled to paid time off work for the appointment.

WHAT IT INVOLVES

Asking you questions:
The midwife will ask you about things like your current state of health, whether you smoke or drink, your medical history, and your immediate family's medical history.

She'll also ask you about this and any previous pregnancies.

Doing checks:
Your blood pressure will be checked. You may also be weighed and your height measured.

Your heart and lungs may be checked too.

Doing a blood test:
You'll be asked to give a blood sample for testing to find out your blood group, whether you're rhesus positive or negative, whether you're anaemic, and if you're immune to rubella. Your blood may be tested for certain infections too. You will also be offered an HIV test.

Doing a urine test:
You'll be asked to give a urine sample. This will be tested to see if you have any sugar or protein in your urine and whether you have any urinary infection.

Feeling your abdomen:
The midwife or doctor may ask to feel your tummy to get an idea of the size of your uterus or they very occasionally may ask to do an internal examination.

Planning ahead:
You'll be given your pregnancy notes when your test results are back, if you haven't been given them earlier.

You may be offered a scan (see page 32).

You'll be told when your next appointment will be. Appointments are usually every four weeks until 28 or 30 weeks, every two weeks until 36 weeks, and weekly after that, although in some areas the number of appointments is lower – perhaps a 19th week ultrasound scan and a first antenatal appointment at 26 weeks.

Asking them questions:
If there's anything that's said to you during the visit that you don't understand, or that you'd

like more information about, ask.

Ask any other questions that you have (don't forget your list).

WHERE TO HAVE YOUR BABY

You'll probably be asked early on in your pregnancy – often when you first see your GP to let him or her know that you're pregnant – where you'd like to have your baby.

You don't have to decide straight away. Take your time to find out the information you need to make your mind up. Things to think about or find out about:

• What sort of environment will you feel safest in when you have your baby?

• What sort of environment will you feel most relaxed in?

• What sort of facilities would you like to have available to you? Do you have any special needs?

• What medical carers would you like to have with you during labour?

• What are your partner's feelings?

• What's available in your area?

WHAT YOUR OPTIONS MAY BE

Hospital

Most babies in the UK are born in hospital. Women usually choose to give birth in hospital because they are reassured by the knowledge that there are doctors and emergency facilities on hand 'if anything goes wrong', or because they want to use a form of pain relief that's only available in hospital.

One of the disadvantages of having your baby in hospital is that, unless you're having team midwifery care, it's unlikely that you'll have a midwife you know

with you while you're in labour. Hospitals have standard procedures and policies such as when to start labour if you are going overdue or how breech (bottom first) babies are delivered. You can find out about practices in your hospital from the hospital itself, or from your Community Health Council, or from antenatal classes.

Home

Women who decide to have their babies at home usually feel that they'll be more relaxed and comfortable there. They're often also keen to avoid medical procedures. Another benefit of being at home is that you'll have a midwife you know with you.

The main disadvantage to home birth is usually seen as not having emergency facilities immediately on hand. However, research shows that for healthy women who've had normal pregnancies, the risks are minimal.

Remember if at any point you change your mind about where you'd like to have your baby, you can make new arrangements.

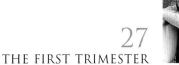

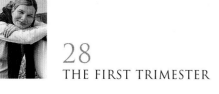

TALKING TO PROFESSIONALS

Jot down some notes to help you remember all the points you want to cover at each appointment with your carers. You'll probably find there's a lot you'd like to discuss.

Many of us are in awe of medical professionals. We see them as being the experts and feel that we can't question what they say. They *are* experts, but that doesn't mean that you can't ask them questions or express a different point of view. You're an expert too – about your own wishes, feelings and needs. If there's anything troubling you about your antenatal care, don't keep worries to yourself.

THE RIGHT TO KNOW

As someone who's being given medical care, you have the right to information about that care. You also have the right to accept or refuse any procedures, treatment or tests that are offered to you as part of it. You don't have to agree to anything that you don't understand or are unhappy about.

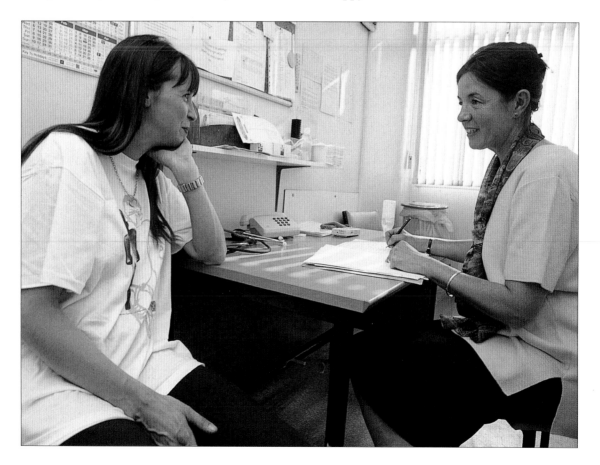

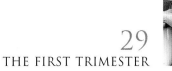

Research shows that women feel more positive about the care they receive in pregnancy if they feel that they've fully taken part in making decisions about it. This means both understanding what is being said to you and getting your point of view across.

When your midwife or doctor fills in your notes, they'll use a set of abbreviations. This is quick and convenient for them, but can be bewildering for you. See page 33 for a list of common abbreviations and what they mean. Ask your midwife about any concerns.

MAKING COMMUNICATION EASIER	
Problem	**Solution**
You don't understand what's being said to you	• Ask for it to be explained. Keep asking until you're able to repeat what's been said to you in your own words. Then ask if what you've just said is right
You feel 'small' and powerless talking to medical professionals	• Help yourself feel more confident by treating them as your equal. Use their name (if they use your first name, use theirs). Get onto the same level as them (sit up if you've been lying down, or ask them to sit if they've been standing). If you've taken any clothes off, cover yourself up. Remember that who you're talking to is a person, just as you are
You're nervous about talking to professionals	• Make yourself as well-informed as you can in advance. Read books and magazines, go to antenatal classes, talk to other women • Prepare yourself by practising what you want to say in advance, with your partner or in front of a mirror • Make notes and take them with you • Relax. Take a deep breath (or two or three), drop your shoulders, loosen your jaw, stretch out your fingers • Take someone with you for moral support
You don't know whether or not you want to agree to something that's being suggested to you	• Ask BRAN (What are the **Benefits** of what's being suggested? What are the **Risks** attached to it? Are there any **Alternatives**? What would happen if you did **Nothing**?) • Play for time. Ask if you really need to make a decision immediately. What would happen if you left it for a while?
You don't want to agree to something that's being suggested to you	• Say that you appreciate their point of view, but repeat your own. Acknowledge that you understand the possible consequences of your decision • Express your point of view calmly and in a friendly way, using 'I' statements ('I would rather not because…') • Be prepared to compromise if you're given new information that makes you change your mind

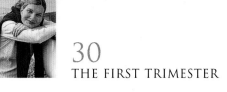

ANTENATAL TESTS

Antenatal testing is a complex area and doesn't always reassure you. You might feel that you don't want to have any tests at all. This is a perfectly reasonable decision to make.

SCREENING TEST

A screening test tells you what your risk is of having a baby with a condition such as Down's syndrome (not whether your baby actually has this condition).

DIAGNOSTIC TEST

A diagnostic test tells you for certain whether your baby has a condition such as Down's syndrome or spina bifida.

GENETIC CONDITION

Conditions such as Down's, Edward's and Turner's syndromes are the result of faulty genetic information in either the egg or the sperm that fused to make the baby. So genetic conditions are built into the baby from the moment of conception and they cannot be corrected.

CONGENITAL CONDITION

Congenital conditions are the result of something going wrong while the baby is growing inside the womb. With spina bifida, the membranes and bones that should grow over the spinal cord to protect it fail to develop, so that the nerves are exposed and easily damaged. Other congenital abnormalities can be caused by a viral or bacterial infection in the womb.

If you wouldn't under any circumstances consider a termination, and you don't feel the need to know whether your unborn baby has any genetic or developmental problems, you can refuse the tests that will be offered to you. If you do decide to go ahead, the first thing you need to understand is the difference between screening and diagnostic tests. There is also a difference between genetic and congenital conditions (see box on left). Here, we list the times when tests will be offered to you and the form each test takes.

10 TO 13 WEEKS OF PREGNANCY

Chorionic Villus Sampling (diagnostic)
Chorionic Villus Sampling (CVS) can tell you whether your baby has a genetic condition such as Down's syndrome, but not whether she will have a congenital condition such as spina bifida. It is the only diagnostic test which is widely available to women before 14 weeks of pregnancy. There is a 0.5 to 2% risk of miscarriage following the procedure, which is an important factor to take into account when deciding whether or not you want to have the test. The procedure involves taking a tiny sample of the placenta by inserting a fine needle through the wall of your abdomen. Ultrasound scanning helps the doctor position the needle correctly. The sample is sent away to a medical laboratory for examination and you should receive the results within 7 to 10 days.

Nuchal Translucency Test (screening)

This test has only recently been developed and is not available everywhere. You can have it done privately for about £80 (ask your GP for details). A thin layer of fluid between two folds of skin at the back of your baby's neck is measured using a 'state of the art' ultrasound scanner. Babies who have Down's syndrome (and some less common genetic conditions) have a thicker layer of fluid than unaffected babies. Research suggests that the test is very good at predicting which women are at the highest risk of being pregnant with Down's syndrome babies although it is more accurate for women over 35 years, and less so for younger women.

16 TO 20 WEEKS OF PREGNANCY

Blood Tests (screening)

The blood tests that are carried out between 16 and 18 weeks of your pregnancy are screening tests for Down's syndrome and spina bifida and will only be accurate if you know for certain how many weeks pregnant you are. Your blood may be tested for up to three different substances or 'markers', depending on how sophisticated the test is which your hospital provides. Sometimes, a fourth marker is added. Most women nowadays have a 'double' or 'triple' test which means that two or three markers are being looked at.

If you are expecting twins these tests won't be available. It's hard to check for Down's syndrome because the doctor has to be able to test each baby separately. Your options are to have the nuchal translucency test very early in your pregnancy, or to have an amniocentesis later on (see below).

If your blood test shows that your risk of being pregnant with a baby who has Down's syndrome is less than 1 in 250, your result will be described as *screen negative*. This does not

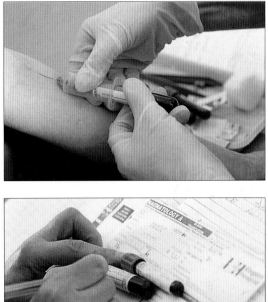

mean that you definitely aren't pregnant with a baby who has Down's syndrome. It only means that it's very unlikely that your baby has Down's syndrome.

If your blood test shows that your risk of being pregnant with a baby who has Down's syndrome is more than 1 in 250, your result will be described as *screen positive*. This does not mean that you definitely are pregnant with a baby who has Down's syndrome. In fact, the likelihood of your baby having Down's syndrome is still very low, but you will need to have a diagnostic test such as amniocentesis to be sure.

Amniocentesis (diagnostic)

Amniocentesis is normally carried out at about 20 weeks of pregnancy, although a few hospitals offer it much earlier (before 14 weeks). Like CVS, the procedure involves using ultrasound scanning to guide a long needle through the wall of your abdomen into your womb from where about 20ml of amniotic fluid is withdrawn. For most women, an amniocentesis is nerve-wracking, but not uncomfortable. You might feel a slight push as the needle goes in.

There is a very small risk (now less than 1%) of miscarriage following amniocentesis, and you will be advised to rest for a couple of days. The results take anything from a week to three weeks to come through. This is a very difficult time when most women feel quite unable to concentrate on anything else except worrying about whether their baby will be OK.

THROUGHOUT PREGNANCY...

Ultrasound Scans (screening/diagnostic)

Scans are useful for dating pregnancies and for indicating whether your baby has developed normally. However, they don't pick up everything. For example, at least 30% of babies with heart problems are not diagnosed on scans. The accuracy of scans depends on the skill of the sonographer, the quality of the machinery she is using, and the length of time for which you are scanned. Scans can identify different things at different stages of pregnancy. If there is any

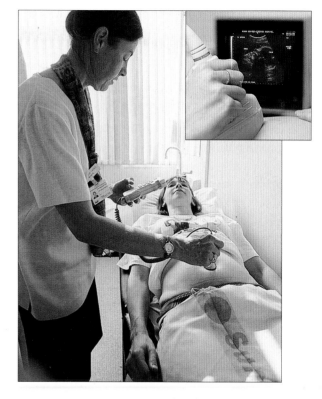

doubt about your dates, for example, a dating scan will show how many weeks advanced your pregnancy is. These scans are usually done at around the three-month mark and certainly before 20 weeks. An anomaly scan to check that all is well is always offered at around 19 weeks.

Weeks of pregnancy	What the scan might show
up to 13 weeks	– how many weeks pregnant you are – how many babies there are – whether your baby's heart is beating – very major problems with the way your baby's body and limbs have developed
18–22 weeks	– spina bifida and hydrocephalus – major heart and kidney problems – problems with your baby's stomach and digestive tract
30 weeks and later	– minor problems such as cleft lip... – some heart problems missed at the 20 weeks scan – minor kidney problems

UNDERSTANDING YOUR NOTES

There is currently no standard format for notes. Their layout, and the information they contain, varies between health authorities and between hospitals.

Abbreviation	What it means	Abbreviation	What it means
Alb	*Albumin:* a protein that may be present in your urine	NH	*Not heard*
Br	*Breech:* your baby is lying bottom down	NF	*Not felt*
		Nil	*None found:* normal
C Ceph	*Cephalic:* your baby is lying head down	NW	*Not weighed*
E Eng	*Engaged:* your baby's head has moved down into your pelvis ready for birth	OA	*Occipito anterior:* baby lying head down facing your back
		Oed	*Oedema:* swelling
		OP	*Occipito posterior:* baby lying head down facing your front
EDD	*Estimated date of delivery:* the date your baby is due	Para 0	*Parity (having given birth):* no previous births
F	*Felt:* movements	Para 1, 2, 3 (etc.) + 1	*Parity:* 1, 2 or 3 (etc.) previous births. Number after the + refers to pregnancies not ending in a live birth
Fe	*Iron:* you've been prescribed iron		
FHH	*Fetal heart heard:* carer has heard baby's heart beating		
FHNH	*Fetal heart not heard:* carer hasn't heard baby's heart beating yet	Prot	*Protein*
		ROA	*Right occipito anterior:* baby lying head down on your right side facing your back
FMF	*Fetal movements felt:* carer has felt baby's movements		
FMNF	*Fetal movements not felt:* carer hasn't felt baby's movements	ROP	*Right occipito posterior:* baby lying head down on your right side facing your front
H	*Fetal heart heard*		
LMP	*Last menstrual period:* first day of your last period before you became pregnant	tr	*Trace:* a slight indication *Transverse:* baby lying sideways across your uterus
LOA	*Left occipito anterior:* baby is lying head down on your left side facing your back	Vx	*Vertex:* baby lying head down
		+, ++, +++	*Indication of amount found:* more plus signs equals more found
LOP	*Left occipito posterior:* baby is lying head down on your left side facing your front	1/5, 2/5, 3/5, 4/5	*Indication of how far baby's head moved into pelvis.* 2/5 can mean two-fifths of head above pelvis or two-fifths moved into pelvis
NAD	*No abnormality detected:* normal		
NE, NEng, Not Eng	*Not engaged:* baby's head hasn't yet moved down into pelvis		

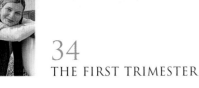
ANTENATAL EXERCISES

You'll probably cope more easily with the physical demands of a long labour if you're fit. Regular physical activity such as brisk walking and some simple movements are all it takes.

If you're not used to exercising, then pregnancy is a good opportunity to start. There are many long-term health benefits – it will help you cope with the increasing demands of growing and carrying your baby and will help you get back into shape after the birth more easily. Start gradually and build up slowly. It's important to choose an activity you enjoy and

getting together with other pregnant women can be a good motivator. Exercising two to three times a week or a good 15–20 minute daily walk is better than going to one strenuous class infrequently.

If you are used to taking part in sport, regularly visit the gym or take part in an exercise class, there is no reason why you shouldn't continue during your pregnancy with a few simple modifications. You'll probably taper off your level of exercise automatically as your pregnancy advances.

Doing exercises correctly is vital to avoid stressing vulnerable joints. Check your posture continuously and try to avoid sudden changes of direction and twisting movements.

If you work out with weights in a gym, pay extra attention to technique and stability. As the pregnancy progresses you may like to reduce the weights and increase the repetitions instead, but do avoid fatigue.

Don't lie flat on your back after the first three to four months of your pregnancy as the weight of the growing baby and uterus can press on the large blood vessels and could diminish blood flow to the uterus.

STANDING WELL

As your pregnancy advances, the growing uterus and enlarging abdomen tend to tip the pelvis forward, leading to an increased curve in the lower back and rounded shoulders. This can lead

SAFETY GUIDELINES:

- Start slowly, build up gradually.
- Exercise regularly.
- Avoid hot and humid conditions.
- Drink plenty of water before, during and after your exercise session.
- Stay aware – you should be breathing harder than normal but still be able to carry on a conversation.
- If you feel faint, weak, sick, or start to sweat profusely or have abdominal pains, gradually slow down and stop what you are doing. Check with your midwife or doctor before resuming any exercises.
- Avoid high impact exercises which involve having both feet off the ground together such as jumping/jogging.
- Avoid sudden changes of direction and pay attention to technique.
- If you have an existing medical condition or have had any problems with this pregnancy, please consult your midwife or doctor before starting exercises.

to muscle imbalance and backache with some muscles being stretched and others shortening. Becoming aware of how you stand and sit during everyday activities can help you to correct your posture and avoid some of these problems.

Stand with both feet hip-width apart and keep your knees straight but soft (i.e. not locked).

Pull your abdominal muscles in, trying to bring your tummy button nearer to your spine (use your muscles to 'hug your baby close').

Lift up out of your ribcage trying to make a little more space between your hip bones and your lower ribs ('think yourself taller').

Keep your chin tucked in and the back of your neck long so that your head feels comfortably balanced on relaxed shoulders.

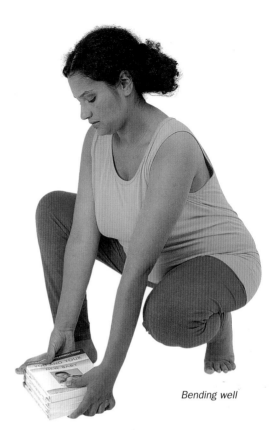

Bending well

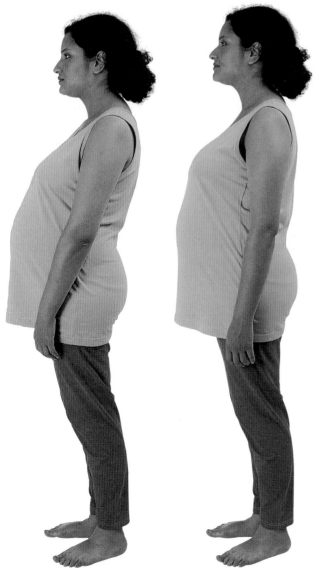

BENDING WELL

If you have to bend down to lift things off the floor, try to keep your back straight and use your strong leg muscles to help by bending at the knees. Keep feet apart to give yourself a wide, stable base and bring the object you are lifting close to your body before straightening up to standing. Try to avoid bending from the waist without bending your knees.

SITTING WELL

Sit in a chair with both feet firmly on the ground. Make sure that your weight is evenly distributed on both 'sitting bones' and that your back is supported in its normal curve. Sitting cowboy-style leaning forwards over cushions on the back of a dining room chair can be very comfortable.

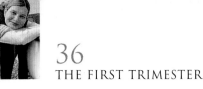
LEG SQUATS

This exercise is useful for strengthening your leg muscles and will help with climbing stairs and lifting.

Holding on to a chair, stand with feet hip-width apart and one foot approximately 30cm in front of the other.

Bend both knees and lower your body until the back knee is a few inches off the floor, then raise yourself up again to the starting position.

Repeat 6 to 8 times and then change legs.

Try to keep each knee as near to a right angle as possible when bending.

GETTING ON TO ALL FOURS

Whenever you have to get down on to the floor safely, use the above movement. This time, however, lower yourself into a half kneeling position (just one knee on the floor) then down to kneeling on both knees. Slide your hands down your thighs and on to the floor so that you end up on all fours. Reverse this procedure to get up safely.

Leg squats

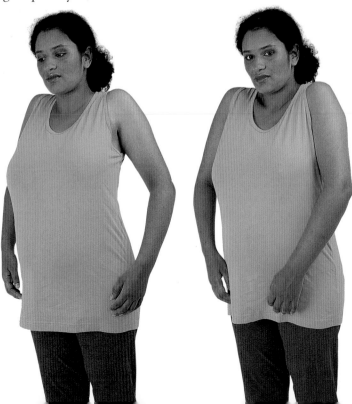

SHOULDER ROLLS

Simple shoulder shrugging and circling (6 to 8 times each shoulder) can stop aching in the shoulders, neck and upper back.

Move slowly and rhythmically, to music if you like, lifting your shoulders up, back, down and round, in large circles. Keep your chin tucked in and neck long.

TUMMY STRENGTHENERS

During pregnancy your abdominal muscles lengthen and widen to make space for the growing baby. If you exercise these muscles during pregnancy, it will help to prevent aches in your back and ribcage, and you should get back into shape more easily after the birth.

Remember that there are four different layers in your abdominal muscles and it's important to work them all especially the deepest layer, the tranversus muscle.

Get onto all fours (see facing page) and exercise the tranversus by pulling your tummy button in towards your spine without moving your back or tilting your pelvis.

Get your partner to check that your back isn't moving while you pull in the abdominal muscles. Repeat about 6 to 8 times holding your tummy in for a few seconds each time. Keep breathing normally.

DO NOT let your back sag while you do this or it may aggravate any backache you have.

PELVIC FLOOR EXERCISES

Our pelvic floor muscles hold all the abdominal contents in place and keep us continent (that is, they stop urine and faeces escaping when we cough, laugh, sneeze or lift). Exercising them now will help prevent problems later.

Imagine you are desperate to empty your bladder but when you get to the lavatory it's occupied. Instinctively, you will do a pelvic floor contraction and squeeze to stop wetting yourself.

Try doing it now – pulling up around the front passage as if to stop yourself leaking, hold for a count of four and then release. You should feel the difference when you let go.

Repeat the exercise in batches of 6 to 8 as often during the day as you can, wherever you are. As well as holding for a count of four, try doing some where you squeeze, release, squeeze, release quite quickly.

Remember to keep breathing normally throughout.

Once a week, sitting on the loo, you can try to stop in midstream while weeing to check that you are doing the exercise correctly but DO NOT do the exercises regularly while trying to empty your bladder as this may increase your chance of a urinary infection.

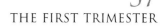

Tummy strengtheners

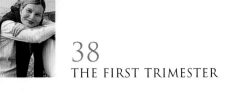

PREGNANCY SICKNESS

Nearly 80% of women suffer pregnancy sickness during the early weeks of pregnancy. It is often called morning sickness although it can strike at any time of the day.

Some women will just feel a bit nauseous. Others will feel sick every day and may actually vomit. An unlucky few will be so unwell that they need to take time off work. The good news is that most women start to feel a lot better around 14 weeks of pregnancy.

Perhaps it would help if we knew exactly what caused pregnancy sickness! Unfortunately, all we have at present are theories – and a few ideas that may help relieve the awfulness for some people, some of the time.

WHY – OH WHY?

Pregnancy sickness may be caused by hormonal changes. The pattern of sickness generally seems to follow the ebbs and flows of human chorionic gonadotrophin (HCG). This hormone orchestrates the production of other pregnancy hormones. Levels rise rapidly during the first 6 weeks, peak at 8 to 10 weeks, and begin to fall at 11 to 13 weeks.

Other pregnancy hormones may also contribute to pregnancy sickness. Progesterone tends to slow down the movement of your gut, so you feel fuller for longer after eating. This may add to your nausea. (On the other hand, the slow movement of food means there is more time for nutrients to be absorbed.)

Some people think that pregnancy sickness may be nature's way of protecting the baby from harmful substances at a crucial time in her development. Many women also develop a sudden dislike of certain foods and smells very early in pregnancy – coffee, alcohol, cigarettes and petrol fumes are common examples.

Although your baby is still very tiny, enormous changes are already happening. These changes take energy. Most women find that it helps to keep their blood sugar levels high. In other words, eating helps relieve their sickness. Pregnancy sickness may be a sign that your body needs more, not less, food. All very confusing!

WHAT ABOUT MY BABY?

It is natural to worry about the effect of pregnancy sickness on your baby. The chances are that she will do just fine. Even if you are sick several times a day, and only eating occasionally, she will continue to grow and develop using energy and nutrients from stores within your body.

Bizarre as it may seem, sickness seems to be a normal part of a healthy pregnancy. There is some evidence that women who feel sick are less likely to miscarry.

WHEN SHOULD I WORRY?

Contact your doctor or midwife if:
• You feel so sick that you cannot drink anything at all, even water.
• You are passing only small amounts of dark-coloured urine.
• You have a fever.

HEARTBURN

Pregnancy sickness does get better – but it may be replaced later by heartburn.

Heartburn is an unpleasant burning sensation in your oesophagus (gullet), felt at intervals during the day and night. It is often worse when you have eaten, or are lying down.

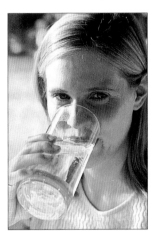

About half of all pregnant women get heartburn. Most find it gets better within hours of giving birth.

Heartburn is caused by small amounts of stomach acid leaking from the top opening of the stomach. The muscle controlling this opening is usually tightly closed, but it becomes looser under the effects of pregnancy hormones. Upwards pressure from your growing baby adds to the problem.

COMBATING HEARTBURN

- Avoid eating and drinking at the same time.
- Eat six small meals, rather than two or three large ones.
- Avoid eating late at night.
- Avoid fatty foods.
- Dairy produce may help – plain yoghurt or a glass of semi-skimmed milk.
- Bend your knees and crouch down to pick things up (instead of bending over).
- Try sleeping propped up in your bed on several firm pillows.
- Ask your midwife or GP to prescribe or recommend an antacid drug.
- Ask a qualified herbalist about safe herbal remedies.

ANTI-SICKNESS TIPS

- Keep eating! Little and often – anything (within reason) that you fancy. Some women are really helped by sucking lemons or peppermints, others swear by crisps, bananas or breakfast cereals. Don't worry about eating a balanced diet for a few weeks – there's plenty of time for that later. Eat something at night if you wake up. It may stop you feeling quite so sick first thing in the morning.
- Rest as much as you can. Can you change your working hours for a few weeks? Could you put your feet up and snooze at lunchtime? Can you use more convenience foods for a while to cut down on evening chores? How about going to bed earlier?
- Find something that helps you with morning sickness, for example, dry toast, plain biscuits or home-made popcorn.
- Try ginger. Many women are really helped by eating ginger, in one form or another. Try ginger biscuits or ginger beer (lots of sugar, so good for energy levels, too). Make ginger tea by infusing a little grated ginger root in a teapot. Add lemon or honey to taste, and drink hot or cold. Try crystallised ginger (often sold in jars of syrup).
- Drink plenty of water so you don't get dehydrated.
- Ask your midwife or GP about taking a supplement of vitamin B_6 with magnesium. This may help if you are vomiting a lot. Foods rich in B_6 include cereals, bananas, baked potatoes, lentils and tinned fish.
- Consider using seasickness bands. Many large chemists sell these.
- Acupuncture may also help. Ask your midwife if she knows of a practitioner who has expertise with pregnant women.

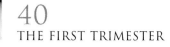
EARLY PREGNANCY DISCOMFORTS

Your baby develops amazingly rapidly, especially in the first few weeks, and all that growth has to be supported by your body. Not surprisingly, this leads to some side effects.

The side effects of pregnancy are what are generally known as the 'minor discomforts'. They are minor in a sense, but if you're suffering from them they may feel quite major, and can be quite hard to cope with. Providing for your baby as he grows is a very demanding job for your body.

Here's a brief rundown of the kind of discomforts you may be experiencing, plus some suggestions of how to cope.

Tiredness
Your body is working very hard to support your developing baby and you may be so sleepy you feel you've been drugged! Pregnancy hormones also cause tiredness. The answer is to rest as much as you can and eat little and often to keep your energy levels up.

Breasts
Your breasts may feel tender and enlarged, and so painful you can't bear them to be touched. Wear a good supporting bra (at night too) and put a cold flannel on them if they feel hot. Gently massaging them yourself also helps, and try cutting out caffeine.

Urinating more often
The extra blood now flowing through your body makes you produce more urine. It can also make your bladder feel full, especially as your enlarging uterus is pressing on your bladder too.

Make sure you empty your bladder whenever you want to, to avoid a urinary infection.

Constipation
Pregnancy hormones soften all your muscles and ligaments which can make the muscles of your bowels sluggish. To counteract this, include a lot of fibre in your diet, as well as lots of fruit and vegetables. Drink plenty of water or fruit juice and relax as much as you can when you open your bowels.

Headaches
An increase in pressure in the blood vessels in your head, due to the increase in circulation may cause headaches. Anxiety and tension can lead to headaches too.

Try massaging your scalp with your fingers as if you were washing your hair. Find somewhere quiet to sit down and breathe deeply for at least 10 minutes, letting the tension flow out of you. Drink a large glass of water and then take a paracetamol tablet if you still have an aching head. Cutting down on caffeine can also reduce headaches.

Dizziness
Your blood pressure may be lower than usual, and if you stand for a long time or get up too quickly, the blood supply to your brain may be temporarily reduced, which makes you dizzy. Dizziness can also be

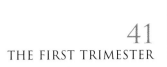

caused by blood sugar levels getting too low. Don't stand anywhere for a long time if you can avoid it and get up slowly from sitting or lying down. Try not to go too long between meals. If you do feel faint, sit down and put your head between your knees, loosen any tight clothing, and breathe deeply.

Stuffy nose, runny nose or nosebleeds

The pregnancy hormones and the extra blood circulating round your body can also affect the lining of your nose.

Treat your nose gently – don't blow it too hard. For a stuffy nose, try a steam inhalation but do consult your doctor before taking any decongestants.

If you get a nosebleed, pinch the sides of your nose gently and lean forward until it stops.

Bleeding gums

This is caused by a combination of pregnancy hormones softening your tissues and the increased blood circulation making your gums soft and spongy. Brush your teeth gently with a soft brush, especially along the gum-line. Use dental floss every day and avoid sugary food and drink. Do try to see your dentist regularly – appointments are free now and until your baby is a year old.

Thrush

Thrush, caused by the fungus Candida albicans, is a thick white vaginal discharge which causes redness and itching around your vagina. Because pregnancy hormones change the acid–alkali balance in the vagina, this makes it easier for thrush to develop. You can help yourself by wearing cotton knickers and not wearing tights; cutting down on sugary foods; eating live yoghurt, and using an antifungal cream or pessary (if you buy this over the counter, tell the pharmacist that you're pregnant).

FEELING WOBBLY?

It's not unusual in early pregnancy to find that your emotions are all over the place. This is partly because of the massive hormonal changes that are happening inside you. But it's also a normal response to the huge change in your life that being pregnant brings about. No matter how thrilled you are, you're probably having moments of anxiety too. You may be worried about being a parent and how this is going to affect your life and your relationship with your partner. You may be anxious about what's going to happen to your body while you're pregnant. You're almost certainly concerned for the well-being of your baby.

The best way of coping with these anxieties is to talk about them, with your partner, or a family member or a friend. Talking also prompts you into taking some action to deal with your worries, which can be a positive help too.

CHANGING TASTES

It's a common notion that pregnant women have cravings for strange things, or strange combinations of things, to eat. Some do, but by no means all. If you're having cravings, there's probably no harm in giving in to them, especially if the craving's so intense that you can't relax until you've satisfied it, but be careful not to eat too many sweet things, and make sure you're having enough fibre.

A lot of women go off certain foods or drink – especially things like alcohol and coffee, and fried or rich food, which aren't very good for you anyway. It may be your body's way of telling you to eat well.

SECOND TRIMESTER 13–28 WEEKS

Your pregnancy is now established and your baby is well formed. Unless you're unlucky, or expecting twins or triplets, sickness will lessen considerably and you should start to feel more energetic.

This is the middle stage of pregnancy when you're supposed to bloom (although you might find that you're one of those flowers that still wilts!).

Brown pigmentation develops on your body. Your nipples and areolae may have already got darker, and you may now develop a fine brown line running from navel to pubic bone. Some women also get a brown 'butterfly mask' on the face, which can get darker if exposed to the sun. As your belly grows, stretch marks may begin to appear.

Inside the womb, your baby now looks like a real human being and behaves like one too, moving limbs and exercising his muscles. Most women feel movements for the first time between 18 and 22 weeks, and then they'll feel like tiny flutterings or bubbles.

At 16 weeks there is a fine growth of hair (lanugo) all over the six-inch long body and at week 20 teeth are forming in the jawbone and hair may be growing on the head. At week 24, your baby can cough, swallow, hiccup and even suck his thumb. His skin is red at this stage and you can see veins clearly. At 24 weeks, he can hear and is becoming familiar with your voice.

By week 28, his body is covered in vernix, a greasy white substance which protects his skin from getting soggy in the amniotic fluid, and he's getting plumper. His eyes are now open, and he can tell light from dark.

The second trimester is a good time to join an antenatal class.

WHAT YOU CAN GET FROM CLASSES

• *Information about pregnancy, labour, birth and the early days with your new baby*
You can of course get information from lots of other sources, but classes give you the opportunity of asking questions, as well as discussing things with other mothers-to-be.

No two pregnancies
are the same – some
babies are bigger, some
smaller and each one
is unique.

• *Practical skills*

In some classes you can try out practical skills for labour and birth. The teacher will demonstrate techniques to you.

• *Involving your partner*

Some classes are for men as well as for women. Going to classes can help your partner to feel actively involved in your pregnancy. If he's going to be your labour companion, they're also a good way for him to learn about what to expect in labour and how he can help you.

• *Planning for the birth*

You can find out from classes what your options are for labour and your baby's birth so that you can decide what you would like.

• *Meeting people*

You'll meet other people who are going through the same kinds of experiences and have the same kinds of concerns as you do, and will be able to share ideas or anxieties. You may make friends too, who can give you support in the last stages of your pregnancy, as well as after your baby's born. Some friendships last a long time.

• *Confidence*

Getting information, learning skills, finding out about your options and sharing ideas with others can all help you feel more confident.

• *Time to focus*

If you lead a very busy life, it might be hard for you to find time to think about the birth and about your baby. Classes give you that time.

WHAT CLASSES ARE AVAILABLE

There are various different types of classes, but not all of them are available in all areas.

• *Hospital classes* are held at a hospital clinic for women who are having their babies at that hospital. They're usually run by a hospital midwife. The classes are often quite large and may be rather formal. There's no charge.

• *Clinic classes* are held at a local clinic, health

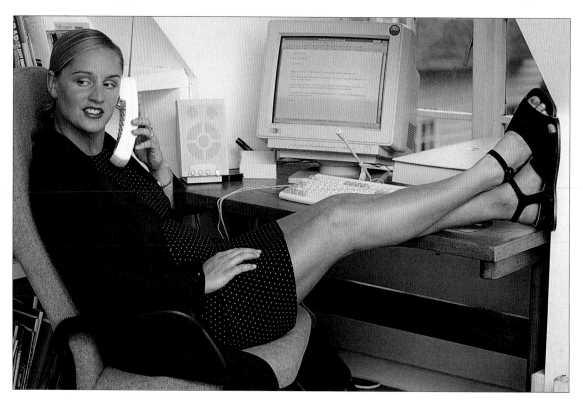

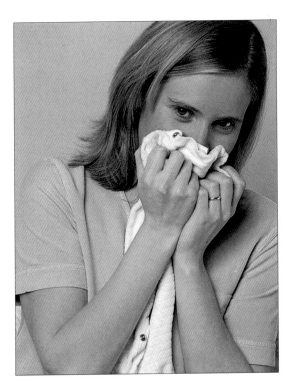

centre or GP's surgery, and are usually run by a community midwife. The classes are often smaller and less formal than the hospital ones, and give you the opportunity of meeting people in your area. They're free.

• *NCT classes* are run by NCT-trained teachers and may be held at the teacher's home or in a hall. The groups are small and informal, and the emphasis is on learning through discussion. The classes focus on exploring options and encouraging you to make up your own mind about them. There's a charge.

• *Active birth classes* are run by teachers who have trained with the Active Birth Centre. They focus on preparing your body physically for labour, with an emphasis on using your own resources in labour. There's a charge.

• *Other classes.* In some areas, there may be classes available at private birthing centres.

Most classes are designed to start when you're around 28 weeks' pregnant, though some start earlier. You need to book them well in advance.

ACTION PLAN

13–16 WEEKS

You can stop taking a folic acid supplement, unless you're advised to continue.

Any screening blood tests you're having will be carried out now (see page 31).

Amniocentesis can be done (see page 31).

Remember to give your employer at least three weeks' written notice of when you intend to start maternity leave.

17–20 WEEKS

You'll probably have an appointment to talk things over with your midwife.

You will probably be offered an 'anomaly scan' to check your baby is developing normally.

21–24 WEEKS

If you plan to return to work, think about your childcare options and make enquiries.

Collect form MatB1 from your midwife. It's your written proof of pregnancy and you'll need it for claiming benefits.

Think about who you would like to have as a labour partner (see page 52).

If you are planning on a waterbirth, hire a birthing pool now.

25–28 WEEKS

If you don't qualify for statutory maternity pay, ask for a maternity allowance claim pack, with form MA1 from your benefits agency. Fill it in and send it off with form MATB1.

Antenatal classes may be starting about now.

This maybe a good time to shop for baby items, before you get too uncomfortable.

Week 27 is usually the last week that you can travel by air without a doctor's note (you can travel until 36 weeks with a note) or without a medical certificate.

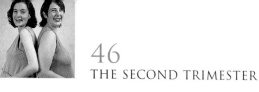

WEIGHT GAIN

Many areas no longer weigh women in antenatal clinics apart from booking in. There's an enormous variation in the amount of weight women put on.

Research has shown that a woman can gain anything from almost nothing to up to 23kg, and still have a normal pregnancy and a healthy baby. Each individual woman's weight gain will depend on her own individual metabolism and her own individual needs.

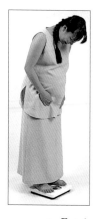

WHAT MAKES UP THE EXTRA?

• Your baby.
• Your baby's support system (the placenta, amniotic fluid, your enlarged uterus, your extra blood supply).
• Your enlarged breasts.
• Extra fluid (needed to make your body soft and stretchy so that it will give when your baby is born).
• Fat (provides an energy store as a back-up in case for any reason you're not able to take in enough food during pregnancy or while you're breastfeeding).

WHY WATCH YOUR WEIGHT?

• The reason low weight gain may be viewed with concern is that it's taken as a sign that the baby might not be growing properly. But as it's impossible to separate out the different things that make up your extra weight, weight gain on its own isn't a reliable indication of how well your baby is growing.
• If you put on a lot of weight, especially in later pregnancy, it may be because you're retaining a lot of fluid. This is quite normal, but it can also be a sign of pre-eclampsia (see pages 66–67). However, this is only the case if you have high blood pressure too.
• Being overweight may make you more prone to certain pregnancy discomforts.
• You may be worrying that if you gain a lot of weight you'll never lose it. Few women go back to exactly the same shape they were before they were pregnant, but weight gain in pregnancy rarely leaves you permanently overweight.

LOOKING AFTER YOUR BACK

Most of the weight that you gain when you're pregnant goes on around your front, and this can lead to you developing the typical duck-like pregnant woman's stance – protruding belly, bottom sticking out, shoulder blades pulled back and lower back curved in. All of this can lead to backache.

Taking care of your back

• Be careful about your posture. Try not to let your abdomen pull your lower spine too far forward. You can correct this by tilting your pelvis (see box).

• Remember that your back was not designed for bending in half. Use your knees instead.

• Keep moving. Activities like walking and swimming will help keep your spine flexible.

• If you rest or sleep lying on your back (though it's better not to once you're into the second trimester of your pregnancy), roll over onto your side before you get up, so that you don't put too much strain on your back.

• Wear flat shoes.

• You'll find some useful exercises to strengthen back and tummy muscles on page 37.

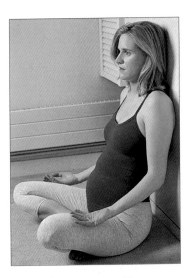

If you're suffering from a bad back try having a warm bath or putting a hot water bottle or an ice pack against your back. You could also get someone to give you a back massage. Try wearing a maternity girdle (if the problem's severe) or seeing an osteopath or chiropractor. You'll find the Osteopathic Information Service in Resources on page 186.

PELVIC TILTING

• Stand with your back against a wall, with your feet hips-width apart and a few centimetres away from the wall, and your knees slightly bent.

• Breathe in, then as you breathe out, press your lower back into the wall. You'll be tilting the lower part of your pelvis forward, so that you're tucking your bottom in (it'll come away from the wall) and pulling your abdomen back. When your pelvis is in this position, your back will be straighter. Also your buttock and tummy muscles will be able to help support the weight of your abdomen, relieving the strain on the muscles of your lower back.

You can also do this movement sitting, kneeling, on all-fours, or standing away from a wall (just imagine it's there).

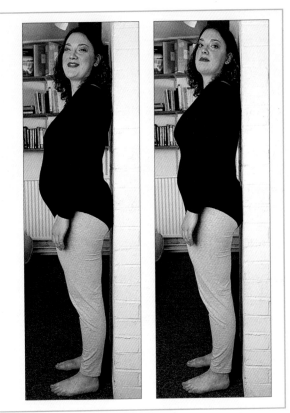

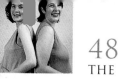

WATERBIRTH

We all know that warm water can be wonderfully relaxing. To labour and give birth in a pool full of warm water is now an option that many women are keen to try.

Warm water helps a woman in labour because it's relaxing. When you relax, you let go and your body takes over, allowing labour to progress. Water is also buoyant, supporting you and letting you move freely. It's easier for you to change your position in water and just 'go with the flow'. If you have any kind of physical disability, this can be really helpful.

CAN IT RELIEVE PAIN?

Research studies on the use of pools have mostly been quite small scale, but some studies have shown that women labouring in a pool are much less likely to need other forms of pain relief than women not in a pool. One large audit showed that most second-time mothers using the pool needed no other form of pain relief while most first-time mothers used the pool plus Entonox (gas and air) for pain relief.

Other studies have shown that using a pool can reduce the need for assisted deliveries, and cut the length of the second stage of labour. And in a third study the overall length of labour was shorter for women using a pool.

The evidence regarding whether giving birth under water will help you get away without an episiotomy (cut in the vaginal opening) is less clear cut. Some studies showed fewer cuts and more tears in the perineum, while other studies show that giving birth in water means fewer cuts or tears altogether.

All the studies done show no difference in the Apgar scores of babies born to women labouring in a pool and no cases of neonatal infection. The pool temperature is generally recommended to be maintained at 36–37°C as there is some evidence that if it is any hotter it can adversely affect the baby's heart rate.

A birthing pool also allows you your own space and may give you a sense of privacy and security. When you are relaxed, your baby is under less stress and gets a better supply of oxygen. A waterbirth is often a more gentle birth, which benefits your baby too.

IS IT SAFE?

You may wonder whether it is safe for a baby to be born 'under water'.

Babies are brought gently to the surface as soon as they are born, but many women use the pool for the first stage of labour and get out for the second stage to give birth.

In some hospitals you may be asked to leave the pool to deliver your baby, although a recent study of 4,000 babies delivered in the water concluded that it was just as safe to give birth in the water as to get out and deliver 'on dry land'.

It would be a good idea to talk the options over with your midwife, find out what the protocols are at your local hospital and put them in your birth plan.

Portable birthing pools can be hired for use at home or in hospital, and some hospitals will

GIVING BIRTH TO TWINS OR MORE

If you have more than one baby, there's a greater chance that they'll be born prematurely (that is, before 37 weeks), although this doesn't by any means always happen.

How the babies are born depends to a great extent on what position they're in. If they're head down, they can be born normally, but if the 'lead' baby is breech, a caesarean may well be needed. Some doctors always recommend a caesarean for a multiple birth. This is something you'll need to discuss with your doctor before the birth. If you have particular preferences, make sure you discuss them.

Your babies may need to spend some time in special care, especially if they were born early and/or are small. If they do, try and be as much involved in their care as you can.

Feeding more than one baby is very time-consuming, and you're likely to need help and support. You can breastfeed, although it may take a bit longer to get it going properly. With practice you'll be able to feed twins together.

Looking after the babies is bound to be hard work and tiring, especially at first, so accept all the help you're offered. But you'll get tremendous joy from it too!

'You know that love you feel for a newborn? Imagine that twice – or three – times over!'

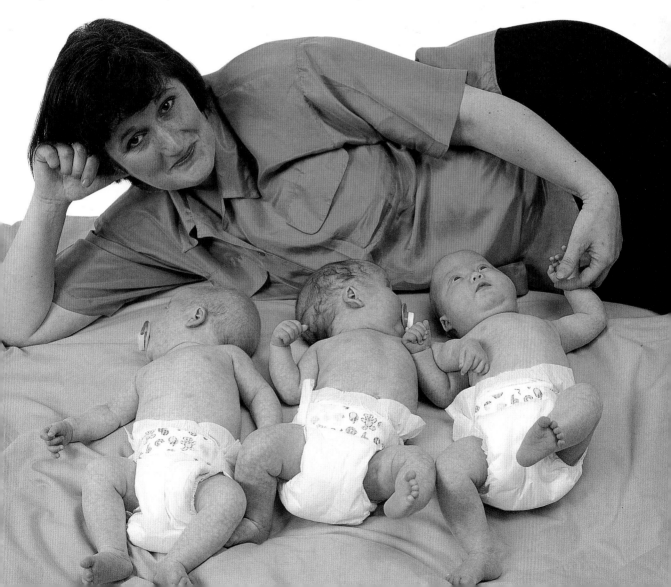

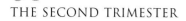

PREGNANCY PROBLEMS

Almost all women at some point worry that something might go wrong with their pregnancy. In fact, the majority of pregnancies are completely straightforward.

If complications do occur in your pregnancy, knowing what to expect can help in coping with them and in making sure that you get whatever treatment is needed as quickly as possible.

PROBLEMS WITH BLEEDING

Bleeding from your vagina at any point during your pregnancy is always a cause for concern. Not all of the things that can cause bleeding are serious, but some of them are. If you notice any bleeding, however slight, contact your doctor or midwife straight away.

LOSING THE BABY

One of the worst things that can happen in pregnancy is losing the baby, and the possibility of having either a miscarriage or stillbirth is every parent's greatest fear. Happily, for most parents, it remains no more than a fear but sadly for some it becomes a very painful reality.

Precise statistics are hard to come by, but it is believed that as many as one in four pregnancies ends in miscarriage.

Miscarriage is the loss of a baby before 24 weeks. Most miscarriages happen in the first three months. After 24 weeks, if the baby dies before or during birth, it's known as a stillbirth.

Parents who lose their baby often have a desperate need to know why it happened, but unfortunately, in many cases there's no obvious answer. This can be very hard to accept.

Losing a baby produces a mixture of feelings – shock, numbness, anger, grief and depression. Although parents who lose babies may eventually come to accept what's happened, they may never get over it completely, and find that feelings of grief well up at any time, especially around significant anniversaries.

An ectopic pregnancy, where the fertilised ovum develops outside the womb, is another form of pregnancy loss, complicated by the fact that it can be life-threatening and future fertility may be affected. A mole pregnancy, where (very rarely) the fertilised ovum fails to develop properly, is another issue again. Pregnancy loss is a complex, multi-layered blow.

One of the things that can help in the grieving process is to see the baby, so that you have someone to remember, even though this may be hard to do at the time, and may not always be possible with an early miscarriage. Another is to talk about what's happened to someone understanding and get as much support as you can – from your family and friends, your medical carers, your religious advisers or a support organisation.

The Miscarriage Association runs a very useful Helpline which can provide support and information on all pregnancy loss. You'll find their details in the Resources section at the end of this book.

The Stillbirth and Neonatal Death Society also run a Helpline, see Resources section.

BLEEDING IN EARLY PREGNANCY

Type of bleeding	What might be causing it	How it might be treated
Slight bleeding or 'spotting' around the time you would have had your period	Your pregnancy hormone levels aren't quite high enough to stop the bleeding, which comes from the lining of your uterus (as it does in a period)	No treatment is needed, but it may help if you rest as much as you can
Slight bleeding after sex	• 'Cervical erosion' (a change in the cells of your cervix, caused by pregnancy hormones) • A polyp (a small harmless growth) on your cervix	No treatment is needed. But check with your GP
Slight bleeding, which may last over a period of days	A 'threatened' miscarriage (a miscarriage that might happen, but in the end doesn't)	You may be told to rest (though there's no proof that staying in bed helps prevent a miscarriage) and to avoid exercise and sex. You may be offered a scan to check on the baby. The hardest part is often waiting to see what will happen
Heavy bright red bleeding, with cramp-like abdominal pains	An 'inevitable' miscarriage (a miscarriage that can't be prevented)	Your doctor may examine you to see if your cervix is still closed. If it isn't, a miscarriage is sadly unavoidable. You may choose to wait at home for it to happen or to go into hospital. You'll probably be recommended to have a minor operation afterwards to make sure your uterus is empty
Dark brown bleeding, with low abdominal pain, between 4–10 weeks	An ectopic pregnancy (one in which the embryo is growing in one of your Fallopian tubes). If this isn't detected early enough, it can lead to the tube bursting, which is an emergency	Consult your doctor immediately. The pregnancy will need to be ended, usually surgically, although if it's detected early enough, it may be possible for an injection to be used instead

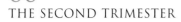
BLEEDING IN LATER PREGNANCY

(Remember that all bleeding should be referred to your midwife or GP.)

Slight bleeding at the end of pregnancy may mean that your labour is about to start. As long as you're in the last three weeks of your pregnancy, there's no cause for concern – just be patient and wait for labour to begin.

Heavy, bright red bleeding in late pregnancy, which may stop and start, could mean that you have a low-lying placenta (a 'placenta praevia'), which is partly or completely over your cervix.

You'll be advised to have a scan to find out whether the placenta is low-lying. If it is, you'll be advised to stay in hospital until your baby is born and your doctor may recommend a caesarean.

However, bright red bleeding in late pregnancy, either slight or heavy, which is also associated with pain in your lower abdomen (your abdomen may go hard) could be 'placental abruption' or 'abruptio placenta', which means that part of your placenta has come away from the wall of your uterus. This is an emergency and needs urgent treatment.

You'll be advised to have a scan to see how much of the placenta has come away and to check on the baby. If the bleeding is slight, you'll be advised to rest in hospital till it stops. If it's severe, and the baby shows signs of distress, the baby will need to be delivered, usually by caesarean.

HIGH BLOOD PRESSURE

A slight increase in blood pressure is quite normal in pregnancy, especially in the later stages. If it goes above a certain level, though, that can cause problems. The main one is that if your blood pressure is high, the supply of blood to your uterus (and therefore to the placenta) is reduced, which means that your baby gets less oxygen. High blood pressure can also be an indication of other problems, such as something wrong with your kidneys. It's also one of the signs of pre-eclampsia (see below).

If your blood pressure is consistently high, you'll probably be advised to rest, to help keep a good supply of blood going to your uterus. As you're likely to be feeling quite well, having to stay in bed might be very frustrating.

For a diagnosis of high blood pressure to be made, a high level has to be recorded over several readings. All sorts of things can make your blood pressure go up temporarily – such as stress, anxiety, or rushing to the clinic – and one high reading doesn't necessarily mean that there's a problem. Try and relax when you're having your blood pressure checked, and if it's found to be high, ask if it can be re-checked a bit later.

PRE-ECLAMPSIA

Pre-eclampsia is an illness which occurs only in pregnancy, usually in the last few weeks. No one knows exactly what causes it, but it seems to be connected with the placenta not developing properly for some reason.

It's possible for you to have pre-eclampsia and to feel perfectly well. The indications that you may have it are that your blood pressure is high and you have some protein in your urine. Another sign is swelling in your feet, hands and face, but this is common in normal pregnancy too. Having any one of these symptoms on its own doesn't necessarily mean that you have pre-eclampsia, but if you have two or more of them, it's possible that you do. A blood test can confirm the diagnosis.

Once you have pre-eclampsia, it won't go away until your baby is born. It's possible for it to get worse very suddenly, causing severe problems both for you and your baby. Severe headaches, disturbed vision and pain in your upper abdomen are all symptoms of advanced pre-eclampsia.

If your doctor suspects that you have pre-eclampsia, you're likely to be asked to go into hospital, so that you can be closely monitored in case things get suddenly worse.

The only treatment for pre-eclampsia is for your baby to be born. This may be problematic if the baby is still immature. The risks to you and the baby from continuing the pregnancy with pre-eclampsia have to be carefully weighed against the risks to the baby of being born early.

THE RHESUS FACTOR PROBLEM

The rhesus factor problem only arises if you have rhesus negative (Rh−) blood and your baby has rhesus positive (Rh+), which he may well be if your partner is Rh+.

The problem occurs because if Rh− blood comes into contact with Rh+ blood, it develops antibodies to the Rh+ cells, which kill the Rh+ cells off. So if any of your baby's blood gets into your circulation, you'll develop antibodies to it.

In most first pregnancies, this isn't usually a problem as generally your blood doesn't come into contact with your baby's until the birth. But once any contact has taken place, unless steps are taken to prevent it, the antibodies you develop stay in your system, and if you're then pregnant again with another Rh+ baby, they can attack the baby's blood, damaging or even destroying his red blood cells.

You'll find out if you're Rh− from tests done on the blood sample that you're asked to give at one of your early antenatal appointments. If you are, the blood is also checked continually to see if you have any antibodies.

Shortly after your baby is born, you'll be given an injection of a substance called Anti-D. This destroys any Rh+ cells that may have got into your bloodstream so you won't produce any more antibodies. If necessary the baby will be treated too.

PREGNANCY-RELATED DIABETES

Pregnancy-related or 'gestational' diabetes is a condition that may develop in the second half of pregnancy. It's termed diabetes because it's characterised by having a high level of sugar in your blood, as in true diabetes, but it's unlike true diabetes in that it doesn't occur because of any underlying disorder and it isn't lasting. It's a condition that develops as a result of changes in your body chemistry and in most cases, it disappears shortly after the baby is born. As it can indicate that true diabetes may develop in your baby later on, stringent control of blood sugar is necessary.

Your blood sugar levels are screened by the urine tests that are done at your antenatal appointments. It's normal for these levels to be slightly raised, but if they're above a certain point, you may be asked to have some blood tests to check blood glucose levels more fully.

If you're diagnosed as having gestational diabetes, you may be advised to monitor your own blood sugar levels, to cut out sugary foods, or possibly to take insulin. You're also likely to be carefully monitored.

The exact nature of the risks, if any, of having high levels of blood sugar in pregnancy hasn't been conclusively established. You may find it reassuring to have these tests and to take steps to control your sugar levels if the tests show that they're needed, as a precaution. On the other hand, you may find the measures worrying. If you do, and would prefer to avoid them, discuss with your doctor whether they're really necessary.

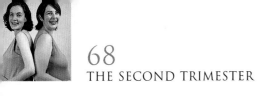

YOUR CHANGING RELATIONSHIPS

The birth of a baby is good news for the whole family, but it does mean adjustments. A newcomer always changes relationships, and the biggest change will be between you and your partner.

SEX – BETTER OR WORSE?

Being pregnant changes most aspects of your life – including your sex life. Some couples find that their sex life is better than ever, while for others it seems to come to a virtual standstill.

- You may be concerned that making love will harm the baby. This is rarely the case. Sex during pregnancy is quite safe for the baby, unless your doctor advises you otherwise.
- Some women feel really sexy when they're pregnant, while others feel too tired and uncomfortable for sex – or are turned off by the baby livening up the minute they get into bed!
- Your feelings about your body affect how desirable you feel. If you love your new shape, you may feel very sensual. It's hard to feel sexy when you're feeling bad about your body.
- As your bump gets bigger, you need to find different positions. This can be exciting – or a turn-off.
- Sex can be great when you don't have to worry about contraception!

Don't forget that there's more to a sex life than intercourse. There are a lot of other pleasurable ways of being intimate.

When you become pregnant, you take on a whole new role – that of the mother-to-be of your new baby. This inevitably has an effect on the roles you have already – as a partner, a daughter, and, if this isn't your first baby, a mother – and you'll find that your relationships will change in various ways.

WITH YOUR PARTNER

It takes two people to make a pregnancy happen, but after that it's a very different kind of experience for each of them. You're the one with the baby growing inside you, you're the one whose body is changing day by day, you're the one who's no doubt having to adjust your lifestyle. For your partner, on the other hand, although a huge change has taken place in his life, *outwardly everything stays the same.*

- Some men want to be as involved as possible in their partner's pregnancy, while others prefer to stand back. Some women like their partners to be involved, others don't. There's no right or wrong about this, but talk to each other honestly about what you want, so that you each understand the other's feelings.
- Many men love their

partner's pregnant shape, and feel very proud of it. Others feel resentful that their partner's body, which they see as having been 'theirs', has been taken over by someone else.

• Your feelings about each other will almost certainly change in some way. Pregnancy brings a lot of couples closer together, and many men say that they feel a lot more protective towards their partners when they're pregnant. But some men feel as if they've been shut out.

• Both of you will have worries about the pregnancy, about the baby, and about your future as parents. It helps if you can share these with each other.

The more you're able to talk to each other about your feelings, the easier you may find it to cope with them, and the stronger you'll feel, both as individuals, and as a couple. You'll also be building the foundations for the two of you as a unit, as parents.

WITH YOUR PARENTS

Your parents may be thrilled that you're pregnant, but their feelings may be rather mixed too.

• They have to adjust to the idea of you as a parent rather than as a daughter.

• They have to come to terms with the fact that pregnancy is a different kind of experience now from what it was when your mother was pregnant with you.

You may be able to acknowledge these issues openly with your parents, but if you can't, just being aware of them can help improve understanding between you.

WITH YOUR OLDER CHILD

If you have a child already, one of your biggest concerns will be how she'll respond to the idea of having a new brother or sister. You may feel torn between wanting the new baby (and wanting your child to have a sibling), and not wanting her to feel jealous and upset, or to have her life disrupted. If your child is still a toddler, wait until you're well into your pregnancy before telling her about the baby. One month is a long time for a small child, let alone nine.

Help her prepare for the baby's arrival by:

• Spending time with other children who have new babies in their family.

• Reading her stories about children with babies in the family.

• Letting her feel the baby and talk to it if she wants to.

• When you're reading or singing to her, telling her the baby's listening too.

• Talking to her about what babies are like and what they can do. Make plans for what you'll do together with the baby.

Your child needs to be assured that her world isn't going to be turned upside down by the baby's arrival. It will be better for her if you keep to her routine as much as possible, and don't introduce major changes – like moving her from a cot to a bed or starting potty training – around the time the baby is due.

THIRD TRIMESTER
29–40 WEEKS

Now you're on the home stretch. You'll be getting bigger every day and your baby is becoming increasingly ready to be born. If he's born at any time after 37 weeks, this is not considered premature.

At 28 weeks, your baby will be about 30cm long and weigh about 1kg. He will be putting on weight rapidly now and will gain about an ounce a day. By week 32, in over 90% of cases, he lies with his head down but some babies keep turning until almost the last moment. His movements will be getting stronger and can be seen as well as felt.

By week 40, your baby's covering of vernix will be decreasing and most of the fine lanugo has gone. He can tell light from dark and can hear and recognise your voice.

As these months draw to a close, you may experience a strong urge to clean, tidy and sort things out. In the final weeks, you may also be getting increasingly uncomfortable, with perhaps breathlessness, swollen legs and insomnia at night. You may also need the toilet a lot more.

You may be experiencing Braxton Hicks contractions, too. These are 'practice' contractions which are strong tightenings of the uterus, which may be quite painful but they'll stop if you rest for a moment (if busy) or get up and do something (if you've been lying down).

Towards the end of your pregnancy, you'll probably start to feel very weary. At 36 weeks Tanya says she's looking forward to getting her body back. 'I've had the world's worst pregnancy,' she says, 'with morning sickness, a heart murmur, a urine infection, gestational diabetes. I've even been anaemic. But I'm finding it hard to believe that this is really going to be a real baby.'

In spite of all that ill health, Tanya manages to look as though she's blooming. 'The fantasy is beautiful, and has kept me going, but the reality? Am I really going to be someone's Mummy?'

'The fantasy is beautiful, and has kept me going, but the reality? Am I really going to be someone's Mummy?'
Tanya at 36 weeks

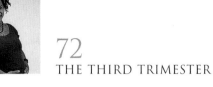
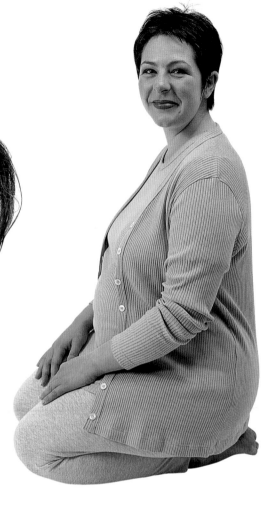

Rebekah, who is also at 36 weeks (you can see her picture on the left) says that she's been wanting to have a bump for ages, 'but I've been quite small all along. People have only just started to notice that I'm pregnant!'

There was some anxiety about Rebekah's baby being 'small for dates'. She feels she was made to worry unnecessarily about this. 'It would've been better if they'd said: this is the problem, and this is what we're going to do about it. But they just sent me for a scan without really telling me why! I phoned the NCT who put me in touch with someone who'd gone through exactly the same experience.

'It really helped me to know that there were other people who'd had the same worries. Now, surprisingly, I've met quite a few people who have said "Oh yes, my baby was small too."'

At any time from about week 36, if this is your first baby, the head will 'engage' or sink down into your pelvis. This means there's more room at the top, under your diaphragm, but may also mean more pressure on your bladder and more frequent trips to the loo. These discomforts can make it hard to sleep and you'll need to find ways of relaxing and keeping your mind occupied.

Things you can do to keep yourself busy in the last weeks include getting a haircut. You won't have a lot of time for hair-care in the next few months so it's worth finding a fuss-free style that suits you. Another idea is to give yourself a long, leisurely manicure and get someone else to do your toes!

ACTION PLAN

29–32 WEEKS
29 weeks is the earliest that you can start paid maternity leave.
If you are having your baby in hospital, ask for a tour of the place where you're booked in for the birth.
Book a TENS machine (from a commercial supplier) if you plan to use one.
Look at what to pack for labour (page 78).
Start practising positions for labour.

33–36 WEEKS
Collect together some basic baby clothes and nappies etc. (page 57).
Get a baby car seat ready to fit in the car
Buy some nursing bras.
Choose your baby announcement cards.
Make a birth plan, with the help of your labour partner and your midwife (page 50).
Stock up on basic food shopping. Buy two of everything non-perishable, so that you'll be well supplied.
Remember no air travel after 36 weeks.

37–40 WEEKS
Make a list of important telephone numbers (GP, midwife, hospital delivery suite) and keep them by the phone.
Have your birth plan and hospital notes ready.
Practise the journey to the hospital in heavy traffic and keep the car topped up with petrol.
If you are having your baby at home make sure you have everything you'll need to hand.
Pack your bags for hospital.
Make sure you can contact your birth partner easily.
Remember that only 5% of babies arrive on their EDD. Plan some activities to help pass the time if you're going overdue.

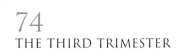
SKILLS FOR LABOUR

Just as your body knows how to breathe and to digest your food, so it knows how to give birth. It will be easier for it to do this if you're working with it, helping it along, rather than resisting.

One of the best ways of helping your body during labour is to relax as completely as you can. If you're relaxed, you make it easier for your uterus to contract and your body produces more of its own pain-relieving substances (endorphins). You tire less easily when you're relaxed, and if you're calm you can communicate better with your medical carers and your labour companion. It's also better for your baby, because he'll have a good supply of oxygen.

Help yourself to relax by:

• Breathing. During contractions, breathe evenly, as deeply and as slowly as you can, concentrating on breathing out. This will help you to let go of tension, and focusing on breathing also gives you something to think about other than the contractions.

• Letting your body flop. Each time you breathe out, especially at the beginning of a contraction, drop your shoulders (your companion can help you with this by putting their hands on your shoulders) and let your body go as much as you can. It is very important to relax at the end of the contraction and conserve all your energy for the next one.

• Relaxing into your companion's touch. Ask your companion to watch for any signs of tension in your body, especially in those areas where you know you tend to tense up (such as your shoulders, or your jaw, or your hands). If they see any tension anywhere, ask them to lay their hands on that part of your body, for you to soften and relax it into their touch.

• Visualising yourself being in a calm and peaceful place, such as on a quiet beach, in a garden or in a cosy room – anywhere where you feel comfortable and relaxed.

• Imagining that the contractions are some other kind of activity, like climbing a hill, or swimming in a sea with big waves.

• Having some relaxing music playing.

USING POSITIONS

During contractions, you can work with your body by using positions that help your labour to progress more easily. However, some people feel they just want to lie down on their side and be quiet in early labour.

BREATHE OUT

Concentrate on your out-breaths by:

• Sighing your breath out, through your mouth, with your lips parted.

• Focusing on something or someone in the room and breathing towards them as if you were sending your out-breath across the room to them.

• Thinking to yourself (or getting your labour companion to say to you) 're-' as you breathe in and '-lax' as you breathe out (or 'let' and 'go') so that you're saying 're-lax' or 'let go' with each breath.

• Going 'mmm' or 'oooh' or 'aaah' as you breathe out.

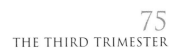

In the first stage of labour

During the first stage your uterus is contracting to open up your cervix and your baby is turning round to get himself into the position he needs to be in for his birth. The kinds of positions that can help with both these processes are:

• Upright positions. If you're upright, gravity helps your baby to move down through your pelvis. Being upright also helps your body to produce the labour hormones that are needed to make your uterus contract.

• Leaning forward positions. When you lean forward, you widen the space between the back and the front of your pelvis, giving more room for the baby to turn. You make it easier for the muscles of your uterus to work too. Leaning forward also helps to relieve any pressure on your back.

• Legs apart positions. These help your pelvis to open up and give your baby more room.

For example:

• Standing up and leaning against the wall, or putting your arms round your labour companion's neck and leaning against them.

• Kneeling up and leaning on a table-top, on the seat of a chair, or on your companion's knees while they sit on the chair.

• Kneeling forward over a beanbag or a pile of pillows.

• Kneeling on all fours (this helps if you have backache) or with your forearms on the floor.

• Sitting the wrong way round on an upright chair (put a pillow over the chair's back).

CHOOSING POSITIONS

If you follow your instincts in labour, you'll find that you'll choose the positions that are right for you. Listen to your body and do what it tells you. Your choice may be influenced by things like:

• Whether you want to be in physical contact with your labour companion.

• Whether you want to have eye contact with your labour companion.

• Whether you want your companion to massage you and where.

• Whether you want to be in a birthing pool, or in a bath or a shower.

You'll be more comfortable if you don't stay in the same position all the time, but keep moving around and using different positions. This will also help vary the space in your pelvis and give your baby room to turn. Ask your labour companion to remind you to change position regularly and to help you to do so.

• Sitting on the toilet – or on a bucket (right way up with a towel or blanket across the opening).

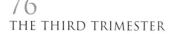
For your baby's birth

During the second stage, your uterus is contracting to ease your baby through your pelvis and out into the world. The kinds of positions that help with this are:

• Positions in which you're upright, so that you're working with gravity.

• Positions in which the back part of your pelvis is free to move. If it is, it will lift slightly as your baby moves through your pelvis, making a bit more room.

• Positions in which you're able to arch your back. When you do this, you make the passage from your uterus into your vagina more of a straight line for your baby to travel along.

• Positions in which you don't feel wobbly. For example:

   • Kneeling up, leaning against the bed or a chair, or with your arms round your companion's neck (they'll need to be sitting or kneeling for you to do this).

   • Semi-squatting, either supported from behind by your companion, or facing them with your arms round their neck, or leaning against a wall. You can also semi-squat between your companion's thighs, with them sitting on a chair.

   • If you need to slow the delivery down (it's better for you and the baby if he's not born too fast), kneel on all fours or with your forearms on the floor.

• If you're very tired, or you have an epidural for pain relief, and you need to be lying down, lie on your left side, rather than on your back.

Massage

Massage is a natural form of pain relief – if you bang your elbow, for example, your instinctive reaction is to rub it. Rubbing or massaging a painful area can also help if the pain is being caused by muscles being tight because they've been working hard or are tense. Massage encourages blood to flow through the area which helps remove the substances that are causing the pain.

These massage techniques can help with pain in labour. Ask your companion to:

• Stroke firmly down your spine with the flat of their hands – this can help you to relax.

• Rub or knead your shoulders – this helps you relax too.

• Stroke lightly – with their fingertips – over your tummy, starting from below your bump (just above your groin), and going up the centre of your tummy, out across the top of it towards your sides, then down each side back to where they started from. This can help if you feel the pain of contractions in your front.

• Press firmly making a tiny circular movement with the heel of their hand against your lower back (at the top of your buttocks). This can help either if you feel the contractions in your back, or if the baby is lying pressing against your back. Alternatively, use a wooden massage roller – or a couple of tennis balls in a sock!

When your companion is massaging you, tell them if you want them to do it more or less firmly, or in a different place.

Keep moving

Moving around is helpful in the first stage for two reasons. It helps make you feel more comfortable, and also as you move you make room in your pelvis for your baby to turn.

The kinds of movement that can help are:
• Walking – either around or on the spot
• Rocking your hips from side to side
• Moving your hips in a circle

Make a noise

You'll probably find that you instinctively make all sorts of noises while you're in labour. There's no need to feel embarrassed about this or to try and stop yourself (anyone in the next room will be far too busy concentrating on their own labour to notice). Making noises is a natural and normal response to labour. It helps you with breathing (if

---

CHECKLIST FOR LABOUR SUPPORTERS ('PURRRR')

POSITION
Is the mother in the best position?

URINATION
Are you reminding her to go to the toilet every hour?

RELAXATION
Is she as relaxed as possible?

RESPIRATION
Is she breathing evenly, and not gasping?

REST
Is she making the most of the break between contractions to rest and refresh herself?

REASSURANCE
Are you giving her constant encouragement and reassurance?

---

you're making a noise, you're breathing out) and with producing endorphins (that's why we say 'ow' or groan when we hurt ourselves). It can also be a way of taking your mind off the contractions and can help you to relax.

Think positive!

Having a positive attitude to labour goes a long way to making it a positive experience.

• As each contraction starts, relax into it and welcome it as another step nearer to the birth of your baby.

• At the end of each contraction, take a big breath out and blow the contraction away – it's gone, it's one more you'll never have again.

• Try visualising your cervix and your pelvis opening up easily.

• Remember that labour is only a matter of hours – it doesn't last for ever.

• Remind yourself what the object of it all is – your baby whom you'll be holding in your arms very soon.

• Tell yourself 'I can do this' – it's true!

WHAT TO PACK FOR LABOUR

As your 'expected date of delivery' draws nearer, start putting the following items into a bag by the front door. Then, when labour starts, you'll have everything to hand.

You won't need all these things. The lists have been made up from the suggestions of mothers all over the country who have found the following items useful to have during labour. If you are planning a home birth, put a few of these things aside in a box or basket so that you'll be prepared when the time comes.

FIRST BAG: FOR LABOUR

• baggy T-shirt or short nighty if you don't want to wear a hospital gown
• thick socks to keep your toes warm

• tissues, hairbrush
• hair ties to keep hair off your face
• toothbrush and toothpaste
• face cloth for wiping face
• two small natural sponges (for dipping in cold water to wet your lips and suck on)
• plastic spray bottle containing water (it gets very hot in labour wards)
• ice cubes to suck (in a thermos)
• Vaseline or lipsalve for dry lips
• talc or massage oil for massage (talc is cooler and drier; essential oil for massage smells nice)
• high-energy snacks (sandwiches, nuts, fruit) for labour companions
• fruit drinks with bendy straws for you
• hot water bottle in case of backache
• ice pack (also in case of backache)
• perhaps an ultrasound picture of your baby to look at
• notebooks and pens to record your labour
• something to do in first stage labour (crossword, jigsaw, magazines)
• candles and matches to soften the labour room lighting
• small change for the telephone
• camera and fast film
• cassette player, tapes and batteries

Keep a bag at the ready and put items in as your due date draws close...

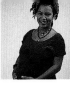

SECOND BAG: AFTER LABOUR

- cotton nighty or pyjamas and light robe, slip-on slippers
- wash bag, make-up, brush and comb, deodorant
- paper pants or stretch mesh underpants
- large size maternity pads (stick-ons)
- witch-hazel for soaking maternity pads in (soothing when placed next to stitches)
- soft bra tops for the first few days
- nursing bra and breast pads for when the milk comes in

Candles will soften the lighting in the delivery room and a notebook will record your feelings

4.00 a.m. First Contractions!

- soft loo roll
- ear plugs/sleep mask if liked
- writing paper, cards, envelopes, stamps, address book, pen
- more small change for phone/numbers on a handy card
- something to read

THIRD BAG: GOING HOME

- an outfit to go home in
- something for the baby to wear
- baby car seat

HOME BIRTH

If you're having your baby at home, your midwife will bring round a delivery pack towards the end of your pregnancy. It contains everything that is needed for the big day and stays with you unopened until it is needed.

You might want to choose a room to use for the birth and get it ready. Clear out unnecessary objects and make sure there's plenty of space. If you plan to give birth on the bed, make sure that it has a firm mattress and put a board between mattress and bed base if necessary. You could make up the bed with clean sheets, put plastic sheeting on top of that and then some old sheets on top, so that when your baby has been born, you can just strip off the mess and go to sleep in a clean bed.

Your midwife will appreciate an area where she can set out all her things.

A large beanbag can be very helpful during first-stage labour – you can lean over it and breathe through the contractions. Failing that, a lot of big cushions will be useful.

If you have hired a birthing pool, practise assembling it and filling it with warm water. It can take quite a long time to get ready. Is your room big enough? Birthing pools vary in size but are generally about 5 feet by 4 feet. You'll need space by the side for the midwife and enough floor space for yourself if you want to get out and give birth out of the pool.

Is the floor strong enough? Large birthing pools hold about 200 gallons of water which weighs about one ton. Small inflatable pools are also available from some hire companies.

...and don't forget your   toothbrush

GOING OVERDUE

Although your head may know that only a few babies arrive on the due date, it's still very hard for your heart not to focus on 'that' day as the one when you should be holding your baby.

A normal pregnancy can be anywhere between 37 and 42, if not 43, weeks long. Calculating when your baby will be born isn't an exact science. It's usually based on the date of your last period, but this relies on you having regular periods every 28 days, which many women don't. An ultrasound scan may give a better prediction, but it becomes less accurate if you have it after about 13 weeks. You'll have a good idea of when your baby is due if you know when you conceived but, even then, babies have a knack of arriving in their own time.

PLAYING THE WAITING GAME

If your due date comes and goes and your baby doesn't arrive, you may be left feeling thoroughly fed up and anxious.
• Arrange a daily activity to occupy yourself.
• Have a long relaxing bath every evening (maybe with music and candles).
• Rest as much as you can.
• If you have an answering machine, change the message to say that all's well but the baby hasn't arrived yet – and leave it on to field the inevitable calls.
• Think positive. Tell yourself that it's only a matter of days before you'll have your baby.

ENCOURAGING LABOUR TO START

• Make love! Semen contains a substance which helps make your cervix soft so that it can open up. Also, when you make love, the hormone which makes your uterus contract in labour (oxytocin) is released in your body and that might trigger off contractions.
• Other things that may help to release oxytocin are stimulating your nipples and squatting.
• Some people believe that getting your digestive system going by eating curry or beans, or taking castor oil, has a knock-on effect on your uterus which makes contractions start, but there's no research evidence for this!
• There are complementary (homoeopathic, reflexology, aromatherapy, acupuncture) remedies you could try. You should consult a qualified practitioner about these.

INDUCTION

Induction is the process of starting labour artificially. Some doctors recommend taking steps to start labour off once you've gone ten days past your due date. Others will wait for up to three weeks. You'll find more information about induction on page 94.

How it's done
There are three steps that may be taken if you're being induced because you're overdue.
• Intravaginal prostaglandin. This may be administered in the form of a waxy-based pessary or as a gel delivered from a syringe-like applicator. The gel helps soften the cervix so

that it can open up, and this can start contractions off. You may need to be given a pessary more than once. Pessaries may be enough to get labour going, but they don't work for everyone.

• Breaking your waters. The midwife uses a long thin plastic instrument with a tiny hook on the end (a bit like a long-handled crochet hook) to nick the bag of waters. This may start labour off. It doesn't always succeed, but when it does, the contractions it produces can be quite strong. It can only be done if your cervix is already slightly open and does not usually hurt.

• A syntocinon drip. Syntocinon is artificial oxytocin, which makes your uterus contract. You're given it through a drip put into your arm. Many women find that contractions produced by syntocinon are very strong and sharp and hard to cope with. Because of the strength of the contractions, the baby's heartbeat needs to be continuously monitored.

These second two steps are often taken together at the same time, with the syntocinon drip in place after the 'forewaters' are ruptured.

What it might feel like

If your labour is started by pessaries alone, it may be no different from what it would have been had it started by itself. This may also be the case if it's started by your waters being broken, though the contractions can be stronger. If you're induced by syntocinon, though, your labour will probably be a different kind of experience. Because of the need for continuous monitoring, you may not be able to be upright or to move around easily. Also, some women find that the contractions are so strong that they need extra pain relief. Even so, if you've become fed up with waiting for your baby to arrive, your relief that you're finally in labour may be enough to outweigh any other concerns!

Making the decision

The decision to induce your labour is a joint one made by you and your doctor. If you'd prefer not to be induced, ask your doctor if you can leave it for a few days. Your baby's heartbeat can be checked every day to make sure that it's normal. On the other hand, you may be desperate not to wait any longer and to get things going as soon as possible. If you are offered an induction, think carefully about the pros and cons. Ask your doctor to explain why it might be necessary. You'll find more about induction on page 94.

If induction is being considered, take your time to ask all the questions you want and get all the information you need before making up your mind.

YOUR LABOUR
AND BIRTH

Labour is a journey into the unknown and no two births will be exactly like each other, even for the same woman. However, there is a sequence of events for your body to follow as it moves through the process.

Nobody approaches their first labour and birth without some idea of what it might be like. There are too many old wives' tales and 'big fish' stories around! Often, the impressions you gain of labour from listening to such stories are rather frightening. However, many old wives' tales relate to times when women were less healthy than they are today, and professional help was more limited in its scope. And you should remember that when women talk about their labours, they tend to exaggerate – not because they have any intention of misleading you, but simply because they need other people to acknowledge just how enormous the experience of giving birth is.

So, listen to other people's stories to find out more about labour, but remember that there is *no blueprint* for labour. Yours will probably be totally different from your mother's or mother-in-law's, or from your friend's.

Towards the end of pregnancy, many women fluctuate between relief that it's nearly over to anxiety about what labour will be like and whether their baby will be all right. While you are going through this maelstrom of emotions, be kind to yourself! If you have finished work, make sure that you get out of the house every day, and have enough to do to keep busy without getting overtired.

YOUR BABY

In the womb, your baby has nearly outgrown the space inside you. At 34 weeks, you were probably feeling him kicking vigorously a lot of the time, but towards 40 weeks, you might find that the kicks have changed to squirming as your baby's freedom of movement becomes more limited. Your body feels very heavy; it's an effort to get out of a chair, to bend down or to

It's mucky and painful and changes you forever. Giving birth means life, and life is a pretty exciting business.

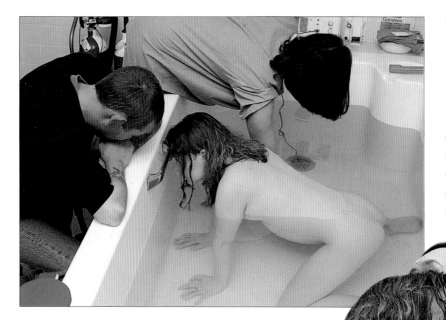

WHAT IS A CONTRACTION?

When the muscles at the top of your uterus contract, they press down on the baby inside and at the same time exert an upwards pull on the cervix so that it opens up. Your body is working hard to push your baby out into a new world.

turn over in bed. Various aches and pains, in your back or your groin, or under your ribs cause you considerable discomfort. Your sleep might be very disrupted because of frequent visits to the bathroom, manoeuvring pillows to try to get comfortable, and sipping milk in order to combat heartburn. If you can't sleep, give in to wakefulness and simply try to rest, perhaps trying the relaxation techniques on page 98.

Before your labour really gets going, you might experience niggly, period-type pains for as long as two to three days beforehand. You might also find that you have a sudden burst of energy and want to spring clean the house from top to bottom. This is quite commonplace. Enjoy 'nesting' and making sure everything is ready to welcome your baby home.

In early labour it may help to experiment with positions to see which are most comfortable for you

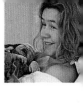

The contractions are a bit like waves. Waves in the sea build up gradually, gaining in strength all the time, until they reach a peak and then crash down on the beach, losing their power and trickling away into nothing. There is then a slight pause before the next wave starts gathering strength.

Birth contractions start as small waves and get bigger and faster as labour progresses. They can be painful, but try to think positively and work with them, knowing that each one brings you nearer to meeting your baby at last.

THE STAGES OF LABOUR

Labour is divided into three stages:
• The first stage is when contractions make the cervix, or neck of the womb, open up to about ten centimetres. Your progress in the first stage is assessed according to how many centimetres your cervix is 'dilated'. This stage is the longest. For a first baby, first stage usually lasts from 12 to 18 hours.
• The second stage is the 'pushing' or 'expulsive' part of labour, when you actually give birth to your baby. It generally lasts about two hours for a first baby.
• The third stage comes after the baby has been born, when the placenta has to come out of the uterus. This stage can last just a few minutes or be over in an hour.

If you think you might be in labour:
• eat little and often
• go for a short walk in the fresh air with a good friend
• gossip on the phone to someone
• find little jobs to do, such as paperwork, paying bills etc.
• get your partner to give you a massage
• have a warm bath or a long shower
• watch a favourite funny video
• tidy your bedroom.

SOME BIRTH EXPERIENCES

Rose's first labour
'It doesn't come suddenly; it's a build up and if you can deal with it mentally and not get too tense, then you can get through the later stages. You can learn as you go along how to cope with things.'

Jasmine's third labour
'It was short and incredibly intense. There wasn't time to think about it or get my act together. It was just happening. The contractions came like a tidal wave.'

Claire's first labour
'Mine was a long labour, a 45 hour marathon. I had lots of time to think. I even baked a pie during the first stage! What I mainly remember is being incredibly tired as I didn't sleep for two nights.'

Palvinder's second labour
'I lost all sense of time from one morning to the next. I don't remember much about some of the labour.'

Louise's first labour
'When I look back on it, I think I had quite a positive labour apart from the last half hour before I started pushing. That was the only point when I said, "Just give me an epidural; I can't take any more."'

Susan's second labour
'It was so fast that I was in shock straight afterwards and couldn't stop shivering. And he was yelling his head off too after he came out. It was as if we'd both been through this big thing together. It was a bond that linked us from the start.'

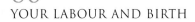

EARLY FIRST-STAGE LABOUR

At the beginning, you might not know whether labour has really started, but when the contractions get going, you will soon be in no doubt that your baby is coming.

The early signs of labour can be difficult to interpret, and you may find that you call your midwife or go to the hospital before labour is properly under way. Don't worry about this. If you are having a home birth, your midwife will arrange to come and see you again later in the day. If you have gone to the hospital, but would prefer to go home again and wait for labour to start in earnest, say so. You don't have to stay.

At the start of labour, the neck of your womb which has been long and hard during your pregnancy will start to shorten and soften, and then to open up in preparation for your baby to be born. Listed below are the signs of early labour and some suggestions about how to cope.

There are three clinical signs of labour:
• A 'show'.
The 'show' is when the mucous plug that has sealed the neck of your womb (cervix) during pregnancy to keep your baby safe in his own environment comes away because the cervix has started to open up. It looks like clear jelly, or might be slightly blood-stained and pinkish. This is normal and all you can do is wait patiently for something else to happen. Labour proper might start in anything from a few hours to a few weeks – it's impossible to say.
• Regular tightenings of your womb.
Some women's experience of early labour is of having long, powerful contractions as frequently as every five minutes. However, this isn't common. You may well find that your first contractions are very mild and infrequent, although they are regular, perhaps one every twenty minutes.

While the contractions are undemanding, rest. Rest should be your priority as you need to save your energy for what lies ahead. It's also very important to have little snacks, perhaps every hour, to build up your energy reserves. Try to relax, following the exercise on page 98.

EARLY LABOUR – HOW TO COPE	
Low backache period-like pains	Wrap a hot water bottle in a soft towel and place it in the small of your back. Curl up in a comfortable position and rest
Sickness	Keep sipping glasses of water, and eat whatever you feel your stomach can tolerate
Restlessness	Occupy yourself with light tasks; try as hard as you can to take some rest

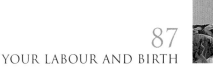
• Waters breaking.

It's not usual for the waters to break at the beginning of labour. They may go with a gush, or just be a trickle of fluid that dampens your underwear. The waters should be clear or straw-coloured. If they are muddy or smelly, this means that your baby has had his bowels open inside the womb, something which can be a sign that he is short of oxygen, although not always. If you think that your waters have broken, phone your midwife or the hospital and tell them how much you think you have lost and what colour the waters are. You will probably find that your midwife wants to come to see you, or that you are invited to go to the hospital for a check.

When to call your midwife/go to hospital

The right time to call your midwife to your home or go to the hospital is when you feel that you would be more relaxed if she were close by. Some people need this security when their contractions are still quite infrequent, and others prefer to labour with just

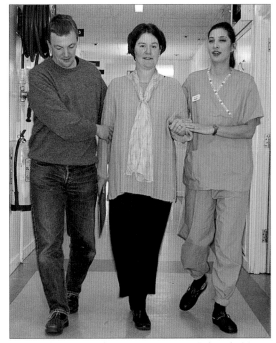

Keep active and mobile in early labour, even if it's just walking the corridors

their partner or chosen birth companion until contractions are very strong and coming at four- or five-minute intervals.

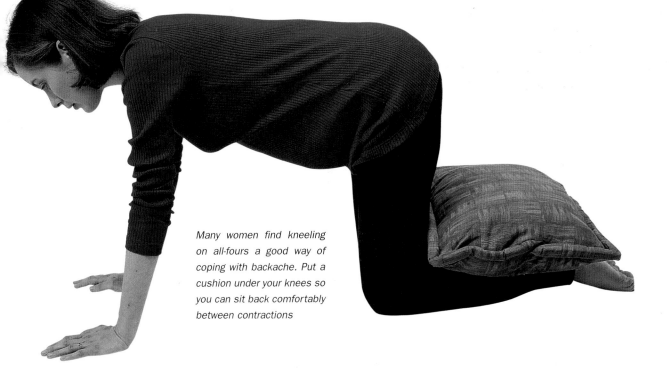

Many women find kneeling on all-fours a good way of coping with backache. Put a cushion under your knees so you can sit back comfortably between contractions

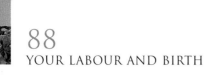

LATE FIRST-STAGE LABOUR

At the start of labour, you will probably feel a whole range of
emotions including excitement, anxiety, joyful anticipation and
fear, but you will gradually begin to focus on the task.

As labour progresses, and the contractions get stronger, you will begin to focus exclusively on what is going on inside your body. You will not want to make conversation or be distracted by having to deal with any practical issues.

WHAT'S HAPPENING?

The contractions are pushing your baby's head (or bottom, if he is in the breech position) firmly down onto the cervix. The pressure of the baby's head causes the cervix to open up or dilate to ten centimetres. This is called the first stage of labour.

As the cervix opens up, your baby's head starts to move deep into the pelvis. The contractions become longer, lasting 40, 50 or 60 seconds, stronger, and closer together, coming at 7-, 6- or 5-minute intervals. You feel the pains mainly in your back, low down, and across your hips, perhaps in your thighs as well. Time starts to play tricks on you, so that hours can fly by without your noticing them, and a minute-long contraction can seem to last forever.

You may feel very serene, confident that your body knows how to give birth to your baby, or you may feel panic-stricken and overwhelmed by the enormity of the experience you are going through. You will probably want to moan and groan and shout. Don't hold back – making a noise is an excellent way of coping with pain! You will want someone to tell you how much longer labour will last, but no-one can give you an honest answer to that question. Your baby will be born when he is ready.

If you are having your baby at home, your midwife will be with you all the time unless you ask her to leave you on your own with your labour companion for a while. In hospital, she will be popping in and out, keeping an eye on you but quite possibly caring for other women in labour as well. If you need her to come to you, don't hesitate to press the bell.

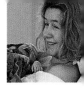
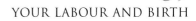

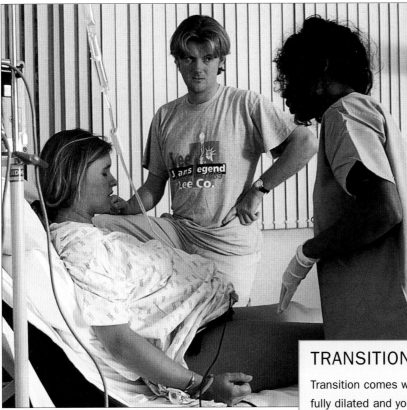

contraction – focus on this contraction, not the last one or the next. Take one contraction at a time.

• The stronger and longer the contractions, the more effective.

• Contractions send you messages about how to make yourself comfortable. Whatever is the most comfortable position for you will be the one that is helping your baby negotiate your pelvis most easily.

It may be hospital policy to give you an internal examination every four hours. If you feel that this would distract you from coping with your contractions, tell your midwife. It may be that she can assess how your labour is progressing by simply putting a hand on your tummy to feel the strength of your contractions and by observing your behaviour. The value of internal examinations has recently been very much questioned in the midwifery journals.

When women are asked, after they have had their babies, which was the most difficult part of labour, they nearly always say the first stage. You feel as though you are at the mercy of the contractions and that your baby will never arrive. Try hard to think positively:

• Every contraction brings you one nearer to the birth of your baby.

• Remember you only have to deal with this one

TRANSITION

Transition comes when the cervix is almost fully dilated and you may feel:

Physically	Emotionally
sick	angry
shaky	abusive
very cold	unable to cope
(especially your feet)	any longer
that your contractions	weepy
have more than	that you never
one peak	wanted a baby
	anyway

If you have been told not to push, it can be helpful to go onto all fours, stick your bottom in the air and put your head down. When the urge to push comes, blow out briskly (as if blowing hair out of your eyes), remembering to pause between breaths. Be guided by your midwife. Some experts believe that telling a woman not to push is unhelpful since the uterus does most of the pushing anyway.

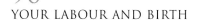

PAIN RELIEF: HELPING YOURSELF

To be able to give birth without pain relief is not to come out top in some kind of endurance test. The tools you need are at hand – choose the one that's right for you.

You have immense resources for coping with pain. Without even thinking about it, you could probably list nine or ten ways in which you tackle everyday aches and pains:

- rubbing the sore spot
- applying heat
- applying cold
- curling up in a comfortable position
- lying down somewhere dark and peaceful
- distracting yourself by keeping busy
- trying to stay relaxed
- holding someone's hand
- listening to music
- taking a paracetamol

Taking a pill is only one of a host of strategies we have all developed to help us cope with pain.

ENVIRONMENT OF BIRTH

Give some thought to the environment in which you are going to labour. If you're having a home birth, you can arrange things as you please, but in hospital, you may need to ask for items such as a rocking chair, or extra pillows, or a large beanbag to help make yourself comfortable. If it's night-time and the lights in the delivery room are very bright, dim them. The hormones which fuel labour are produced more readily when the environment is dark and peaceful with the minimum amount of activity and conversation. Dim lighting will also make you feel more relaxed.

BREATHING RHYTHM

Breathe steadily through your contractions. Focus in particular on the out-breath. Say to yourself '*Re-*' as you breathe in through your nose, and '*lax*' as you blow out gently through your mouth.

Re............................ lax	
in-breath	out-breath
through your nose	through your mouth

Don't let your thoughts wander, just keep them focused on breathing in through your nose and blowing out gently through your mouth.

Even the longest contraction will only last 90 seconds. Your breathing can help you cope with each contraction one at a time. In between contractions, simply rest.

WATER

Warm water gives a lot of pain relief, whether in the form of a bath or shower.

If you have a shower cabinet, you could perhaps try sitting back to front on a plastic chair or an upturned plastic bucket and letting warm water flow over your bump or down your back. It can help to get someone else to direct a strong jet of warm water at the spot that seems most painful.

If you block the overflow of the bath with something like Blu-Tack, you can get a greater depth of water in there. To kneel in the bath on

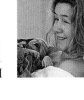
all fours, with warm water surrounding your bump can be very soothing.

CHANGING POSITION

By making yourself as comfortable as possible, you are easing your baby's passage through your pelvis. When your womb contracts, it rears forwards to push your baby's head down onto the cervix and so dilate the cervix. Upright positions make the most of gravity, and leaning forwards helps the action of the uterus. Try leaning onto the back of a chair, or onto the hospital bed (remember you can raise or lower it to suit your height), or kneeling and leaning onto a chair. If you have backache, try an all fours position. Use lots of pillows under your knees and hands to make yourself comfortable. As soon as you become uncomfortable, try another position. When you want to be left alone, bury yourself in a large beanbag and

ignore the rest of the world. (If the hospital hasn't got a beanbag, take one in with you!) If you are upright, try rocking your pelvis round and round, and forwards and backwards. The rhythm is comforting, but rocking also helps your baby's head open up the cervix evenly. If you feel you want to lie down and rest for a while do this if that's what your body is telling you to do.

MASSAGE

Many women find massage helps them cope with contractions. Some don't, and you can't tell whether massage will work for you unless you experiment. Ask your labour companion to massage your shoulders, and especially the lower part of your back. He should use firm, rhythmical strokes, checking with you that the pressure is right and using a little oil to reduce the friction between his hands and your skin.

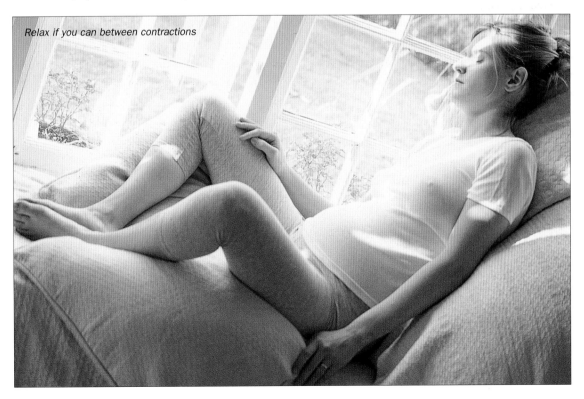

Relax if you can between contractions

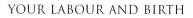

PAIN RELIEF: EXTRA HELP

Here's a breakdown of all the medical forms of pain relief currently available when you need something stronger. They will all help you cope with strong contractions, or get some rest during a long labour.

If you're having your baby at home and you find that labour becomes overwhelming, you could choose to use gas and air or pethidine to help you cope with pain. In most hospitals, you could also choose an epidural. Do check with your midwife whether your hospital provides a 24-hour epidural service.

TENS

With a TENS or 'transcutaneous electrical nerve stimulation' machine, four pads are placed on your back. These are attached to a hand-held control box. Tiny electric pulses block the nerve pathways which carry pain messages to your brain. TENS also stimulates your body's natural painkillers (endorphins). It works best if you start it at the beginning of labour and then turn up the stimulation as the contractions increase in intensity.

Most women find it moderately effective. You'll probably have to hire a machine yourself from a commercial supplier, though, as hospitals generally don't provide them. (Expect to pay about £30.)

GAS AND AIR

Gas and air, sometimes called Entonox, is administered through a mouthpiece or a face mask and, in most hospitals, is centrally

The epidural gives most women complete pain relief and can be topped up as needed

supplied to each delivery room. At home, the gas comes from a cylinder that the midwife brings with her.

To get the best from gas and air, put the mouthpiece into your mouth at the very beginning of your contraction and breathe deeply and evenly to operate the valve. It takes about 20 seconds for the gas to build up in your blood stream and take the edge off your pain. The gas will eventually make you feel a little light-headed and your grasp on the mouthpiece will loosen so that you stop breathing through it and, by the end of the contraction, your head will have cleared.

PETHIDINE

Pethidine is an injection prescribed for you and administered by your midwife. A standard dose is often 100mg, but if you are a very small woman, or you know that the medications you take in everyday life tend to have a powerful effect on you, ask for a half dose. You will need to lie down if you choose to have pethidine as you are likely to feel sleepy once it takes effect. A shot of pethidine lasts about three to four hours.

Pethidine helps you relax and distances you from the pain but it makes some women sick and weepy. It can knock you out so that you 'miss' the birth. It also crosses the placenta to your baby and may affect his breathing, which is why your midwife prefers not to give it if she thinks your baby will be born within three to four hours. It can be useful if you need a rest and are finding it hard to relax.

Diamorphine is used by some hospitals in preference to pethidine and Meptid is another type of sedative sometimes used as an alternative. It may make you feel more sick than pethidine but will have less effect on your baby's breathing.

EPIDURAL

There are various kinds of epidural, and you need to ask your midwife when you see her ante-natally which kinds are available at the hospital where you are going to give birth.

All epidurals are set up by an anaesthetist and then topped up by your midwife at your request.

'Traditional' epidurals involve having a hollow needle placed in the lower part of your back. A thin tube (catheter) is fed through the needle so that the tube lies in the epidural space which is outside the membranes surrounding your spine. The needle is then removed and the rest of the plastic tube is taped along your back to your shoulder. A pain-killing solution is then syringed down the top of the tube somewhere near your shoulder into your back. It feels very cold! You lose sensation from your waist downwards and are confined to bed.

A 'mobilising' epidural involves the same procedure, but the end of the catheter is attached to a pump which administers a small amount of anaesthetic at regular intervals. The degree of 'mobility' varies considerably: some women can walk – others can't get out of bed.

Alternatively, you might be offered a spinal anaesthetic which is a 'one off' injection into the base of your spine. An epidural catheter is also taped into place, but not used as yet. The spinal gives you a couple of hours of pain relief. If you want longer, the epidural tube will be used to top up the anaesthetic in the same way as a traditional epidural once the spinal has worn off.

About 90% of women experience complete relief from labour pain with an epidural, but it doesn't work for everyone.

The disadvantages of having an epidural are that it makes the pushing stage of labour longer and your baby is more likely to need to be delivered with forceps.

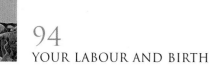

INDUCTION/ACCELERATION

Induction means starting labour off by artificial means. Do make sure that you fully understand the reason why an induction has been thought necessary.

These are some of the most common reasons given for inducing labour:

• Going over your dates

Research shows that, in nearly every case, pregnancies can safely continue until 42 weeks. Babies don't do so well in the womb after this.

• Pre-eclampsia

If your blood pressure is very high and your kidneys are leaking protein, the placenta may not be functioning well. It's safer for the baby, and you, for your baby to be born.

• Baby not growing well or kicking less

Ultrasound scans might show that your baby's rate of growth has slowed. You yourself might sense that she is moving less vigorously inside you. It could be best for your baby to be born so that you and the medical team can give her some extra support.

• Waters break, but no contractions

The bag of waters keep your baby safe in his own world. Once the bag has burst, the baby is exposed to possible infection from the vagina. The risk is minimal in the first 48 hours, but after that, there's a case for induction.

• Genital herpes

Active herpes in your genital area pose a risk to the health, and especially the eyesight, of your baby while he is being born. So if the herpes are in a non-active phase close to your due date, an induction might be suggested to ensure your baby's safe passage through the vagina.

• Previous very fast labour

If you have had a previous labour that took you and everyone else by surprise, you might decide that it would be better to have an induction next time so that you are sure to be in a safe environment when your baby is born.

• Diabetes

Women who suffer from diabetes often grow very large babies. So these women are often offered inductions at around 37 weeks of pregnancy, which is considered safer for both mother and baby.

HOW LABOUR IS INDUCED

The three ways of starting labour are to use prostaglandin pessaries or gel, or to 'break the waters' or put up a syntocinon drip.

Coping with an induction

If you have had pessaries, or your waters have been broken, there's no need for you to be confined to bed unless you want to be. Your baby's heartbeat can be monitored intermittently in a variety of ways, whatever your position, and you should feel free to use all the pain-relieving techniques described in the section 'Helping yourself'.

If you have a syntocinon drip, your midwife will recommend continuous electronic monitoring. There's some risk of over-stimulating the uterus and therefore stressing the baby when labour is induced in this way. Constant monitoring checks that the induction isn't causing any problems.

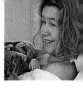
POSSIBLE DISADVANTAGES OF INDUCTION

Induction has its place in the armoury of medical interventions and, when used appropriately, protects mothers and babies. However, it's important that it is not used without a very good reason.

In the 1970s inductions were performed very frequently, sometimes for no better reason than that the mother wanted her baby to be born on a certain date, or the hospital wanted fewer births at weekends! Now, a more cautious attitude is taken, because starting labour off artificially can have its problems:

- The labour might be very lengthy.
- Artificial contractions can stress the baby.
- There is a greater risk of the labour ending in a forceps or ventouse delivery or even a caesarean section.
- An increased risk of haemorrhaging.

ACCELERATING LABOUR

If your labour started naturally and you are having regular contractions, but your cervix is opening up very slowly, you might be asked whether you would like to have your waters broken, or even a syntocinon drip, to speed your labour up. If you're happy to continue as you are, and your baby's condition is satisfactory, tell your midwife that you want to leave things alone. If you do choose to accelerate your labour, remember that the benefits of a faster labour in terms of not getting so tired and seeing your baby sooner, have to be set against the risks of acceleration which are the same as those for induction (see box).

A syntocinon drip can be used to start labour off or to speed up a slow labour

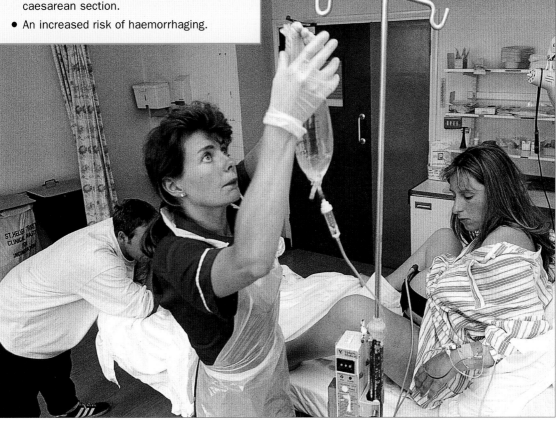

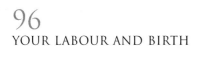

MONITORING LABOUR

Throughout labour, your midwife will keep an eye on both you and your baby. She will use her experienced eyes and hands as well as various instruments.

There are many different ways of checking the condition of a woman in labour and her baby. Your midwife will assess how things are going by how long and strong the contractions are, how you are feeling, how dilated you are and how your baby is managing.

By listening to your baby's heart, the midwife can get a rough idea of how well he is coping with labour. When each contraction ends, his heartbeat, which has speeded up, returns to normal (anywhere between 120 and 160 beats per minute).

There are various ways of monitoring your baby's heart. You are probably familiar with two of these methods from your antenatal checks:

• The 'ear trumpet' (sometimes called a fetal stethoscope or Pinard's) – a piece of wood or metal, shaped like a cone to direct sound waves into the midwife's ear.

• The sonicaid – a portable doppler (ultrasound), placed on your tummy, that acts like a microphone so that you and the midwife can hear your baby's heartbeat.

Research shows that in the hands of a skilful practitioner, both these means of monitoring your baby during labour are as effective in terms of ensuring your baby's safety and your own, as any other.

There are three further methods of monitoring:

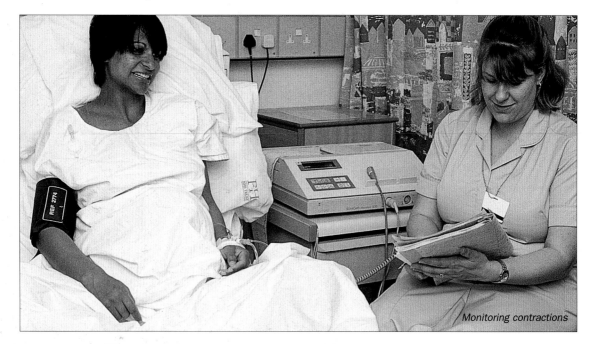

Monitoring contractions

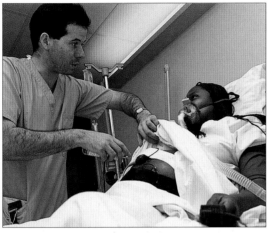

Monitoring labour with an abdominal transducer

• Abdominal transducers

The abdominal transducers are two round discs which are attached to your tummy by belts. One is placed on the top of your bump to monitor how long, strong and frequent your contractions are. The second is placed over your baby's heart to monitor the pattern of his heartbeat. The transducers are linked to a machine which stands at the side of your bed or next to the chair in which you are sitting. A piece of graph paper records your contractions and your baby's heartbeat, and the machine also provides a digital read-out of your baby's heart. Don't be surprised if your baby's heart rate is not steady. This is normal. The readings might well change from second to second.

• Fetal scalp electrode

This is attached directly to your baby's scalp using a metal clip that breaks the skin. It can only be used if your waters have broken either of their own accord, or have been broken by the midwife. The wire from the electrode passes down your vagina, across your thigh to the monitoring machine. Often, an abdominal transducer is used in conjunction with the fetal scalp electrode to record your contractions.

• Fetal blood sampling

By checking the amount of oxygen in your baby's blood, a doctor can decide whether or not the baby is in distress. A little blood is obtained from the baby's scalp by passing a special knife up a tube placed in your vagina. The blood is then analysed immediately and a decision made.

If you have had a difficult pregnancy, and your labour runs into problems, there is a case for monitoring your baby's heart continuously. Otherwise, if you don't want to be tied down, but would like some electronic monitoring, ask just to be monitored for 20 minutes in every few hours with abdominal transducers.

Listening to your baby's heartbeat with a hand-held sonicaid

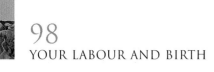

LONG LABOURS

There is no doubt that some labours are more difficult for the woman to cope with than others. On average, a first labour lasts between 12 and 18 hours, but some are a lot longer.

RELAXATION EXERCISE

Rest between contractions as shown here:

- Make yourself as comfortable as possible.
- Put your hands on your tummy.
- Close your eyes and focus on your breathing.
- As you breathe in, feel your tummy push against your hands.
- As you breathe out, feel your tummy fall back.
- Don't let your thoughts wander.
- Concentrate on the rhythm of your breathing.

Remember

- **You are sending oxygen to your baby.**
- Now massage your tummy gently, using circular strokes.
- Imagine your baby lying inside you.
- Relax. Help him relax.

Remember

- **You are both preparing for labour.**
- Continue massaging your tummy for as long as it is soothing.
- Then focus again on your breathing.
- Breathe in and feel your tummy expand.
- Breathe the carbon dioxide out, and feel your tummy flatten.
- Open your eyes.
- Say to yourself that your baby is coming soon. Each contraction brings her nearer.

The length of labour is calculated, in medical terms, from when the cervix is three centimetres dilated. Prior to this, labour is described as being in 'the latent phase'. It's not uncommon for the latent phase to last many hours or even days, and although contractions are generally neither strong nor long, the regular niggling pains that the mother experiences can be exhausting. The midwife might tell you that there is nothing much happening, but it certainly doesn't feel like that to you!

Try as hard as you can to rest during this phase. If you can't sleep, follow the relaxation exercise on the left.

TURN, BABY, TURN

Sometimes labour is prolonged because your baby is lying with his back against yours. He needs to turn right round in order to be born. If your midwife tells you that your baby is posterior (or you know anyway because you have a lot of backache), make yourself comfortable in an all fours position, or leaning onto a large beanbag. Let your tummy hang down. This position will encourage your baby to turn.

Long labours are hard for everyone to cope with. You get very tired and may feel desperate for anything that will assist your baby into the world. Your birth companion may feel frightened that things are not going well. Your midwife is anxious that you and your baby are

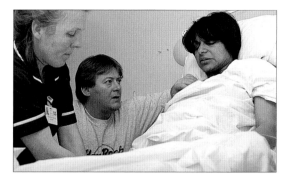

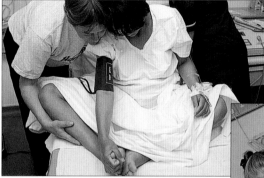

QUICK LABOURS

A very fast labour, when the baby is born within a couple of hours of the mother feeling her first contraction, is not necessarily 'easy'. These labours can be breathtaking for all concerned. The mother is shocked physically and emotionally by the speed with which she is giving birth; her companion and carers are unprepared. Yet babies who come this speedily into the world rarely have any problems – their passage through the pelvis is very straightforward!

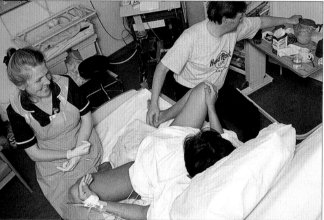

becoming stressed. Yet long labours are part of the natural order of things.

Sometimes, for no apparent reason, the cervix opens a few centimetres and then doesn't dilate any further during many hours of labour. Even using drugs to stimulate the labour isn't always effective. In these cases, a caesarean section is necessary.

MAKING A DECISION

Making a birth plan together is useful because it can give you space to focus on the 'what ifs?': what if labour is very slow; what if it is much tougher than you hoped; what if the baby is in distress and needs to be born quickly? Just thinking these things through together may help prepare you for a difficult labour.

It is important to keep an open mind and make decisions as you go along. If labour is not progressing in the way you expected you may have to make decisions about what is best for you and your baby. Your midwife and doctor will be able to give you the information you need and help you make decisions.

MECONIUM STAINING

A baby's first bowel movement is black and sticky and is called meconium. If a baby has his bowels open in the womb, the waters in which he is floating will be stained by the meconium. Meconium-stained waters mean that the labour requires careful monitoring as there may be a risk of the baby becoming distressed.

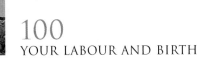

PROBLEMATIC LABOURS

Most of us imagine having a 'text book' labour, that progresses smoothly and steadily. In reality labour varies a great deal from woman to woman. No two births are the same.

We often tend to think of a problematic labour as one in which there is some kind of emergency. In fact emergencies are thankfully few and far between and if you are really facing an emergency the decisions become very obvious. A more typical situation is a labour that slows down or does not progress. Then you may find yourself becoming exhausted and demoralised. You may need to make decisions about issues like accelerating the labour with a drip, or opting for a caesarean, but you usually have plenty of time for these decisions. Sometimes it can be hard to decide and you may need plenty of support from your midwife or doctor.

IF YOU ARE EXPECTING TWINS...

It is increasingly common for women expecting twins to labour normally rather than have a caesarean section. After all, it's hard enough caring for two babies without having to recover from major surgery at the same time! The first stage of your labour will be exactly the same as for a woman expecting just one baby, although if you choose to have electronic monitoring, you will need a special twins monitor to record both babies' heartbeats. Pushing the first baby out into the world is usually not a problem. The second can be more difficult. Because there is so much room inside you once one baby is out, the second can slip round into virtually any position he likes, but he needs to be head or bottom down in order to be born. While many midwives would advocate you being in an upright position after the birth of your first baby in order to encourage the second to get into a head-down position, you may well find yourself on the bed while a doctor checks the position of the second baby and adjusts it if necessary. Your delivery room will be full of people – two midwives, two paediatricians (one for each baby), an anaesthetist in case you have to have an epidural or caesarean, a doctor and perhaps a couple of students. Say if you'd rather not have the students!

IF YOU ARE DISABLED...

If you are disabled, you will already know that you have to work hard to maintain your independence and get the level and kind of care that suits you best. Whatever your disability, it's vital to visit the labour ward long before you are due to give birth, and to get to know the staff. Discuss with them how they can help you in labour. You may have mobility difficulties, but with assistance can achieve positions that will help your baby be born most easily. You may be deaf, and need to remind the midwives that they can communicate with you by writing things down. If your sight is impaired, it's important for you to spend some time in a delivery room so that you can find out where the furniture and different pieces of equipment are. Ask the midwife in charge of the delivery suite

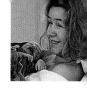
if she can allocate you to the room you have visited or to one identical to it when you arrive in labour.

Your birth companion will be extremely important in helping you achieve the sort of birth that you want. He or she needs to know what happens in labour, and exactly how to help you remain comfortable. Attending antenatal classes together would be an excellent idea.

Just because you are disabled does not mean that your labour has to be entirely managed for you by others. Tell your midwife what you want her to do to help you, and what help you do not require.

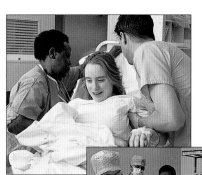

Some labours can be more difficult and prolonged than others

IF YOU ARE DIABETIC...

If you have had diabetes for a long time, you will know exactly how stress affects you, and what it feels like to have a 'hypo' or to have too much sugar in your blood stream. Because labour makes tremendous demands on your energy levels, you will find that your carers (who are likely to include a doctor from the consultant diabetician's team) will want to monitor your blood sugar on an hourly basis. You will have a dextrose drip and an insulin pump in your arm adjusted to reflect your blood sugar readings. Continuous monitoring of your baby's heartbeat may also be recommended. It's not easy to move around when there are so many wires and tubes attached to you. Make sure that the drip, the pump and the monitoring machine are all on one side of the bed so that at least you can turn onto your side. If you have gadgets on both sides of you, your movements will be very restricted indeed.

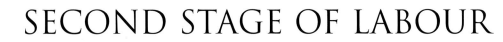

SECOND STAGE OF LABOUR

The second stage of labour is the most exciting part. When you feel the urge to push and you've been told that you can, this means business. Your baby is about to be born.

During the second stage of labour, your baby moves deep down into your pelvis. His chin is pushed firmly down on his chest and his head turns so that the widest part (from front to back) is in the widest part of your pelvis (from your pubic bone to your tail bone).

When his head is being born, you feel a hot burning sensation between your legs as the perineum (the tissue which extends from the back of your vagina to the back passage) stretches. Then your baby's head turns to face your inner thigh in order to bring it back into line with his shoulders which are twisting their way through the pelvis. Your baby's shoulders and body are generally born in a single contraction after the birth of his head.

As you push, you feel strong contractions deep down inside you and a lot of pressure between your legs. You may feel as if you want to open your bowels. This is entirely normal and your midwife will hold a soft pad against your back passage in case a small amount of faeces escapes. Your instinct will be to push, perhaps holding your breath, in short sharp bursts. You won't want to push non-stop from the beginning of each contraction to the end. Nature intends you to push only briefly because your baby's oxygen is diminished while you are pushing and you need to keep his supply going by breathing regularly during each contraction.

Some women don't hold their breath at all while they are pushing. Their breath escapes in grunting noises.

CHEERLEADING

If your labour companion becomes over-excited (and this is certainly the most thrilling part of labour for him, as more and more of your baby's head can be seen), he may urge you to push long and hard, in a way that goes against what your body wants you to do.

Research shows that prolonged pushing and breath-holding do not result in a speedier delivery; in fact, they make you more likely to tear, and are very stressful for your baby. So ignore any cheerleading, and do it your way.

Gravity will help you push

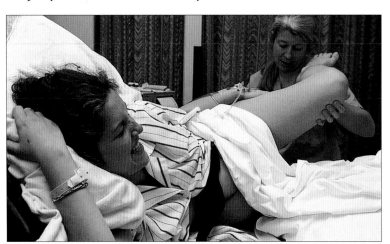

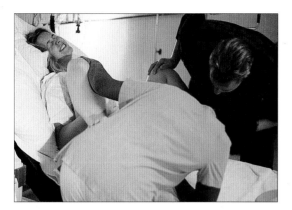

of the effort and be hard work. Sometimes the urge to push fades away and the midwife will help you know when to push. Don't worry if it is taking longer than you expected; try and relax and tell yourself that your baby will soon be born. You may find that it only takes a few pushes and your baby will be born – every woman's experience is different.

THE MOMENT OF BIRTH

How will you feel when your baby is born? The range of emotions is immense, ranging from disbelief that the tiny wriggling baby you are holding at last is *your* baby, elation that you have gone through the labour, relief that all is well, exhaustion from the hard work, worry if all is not well, an urge to just be left alone with your baby, sadness that it is all over, nervousness now that the baby is there and your responsibility. Relax, let your emotions and feelings show – enjoy the moment, allow yourself to switch off from everything else but you and your baby.

your baby out into the world. Lying on your back or in a semi-recumbent position makes pushing harder because the curve of the birth passage means that you have to push your baby up a hill – exhausting for both of you. Try and choose a kneeling position, or a supported squat with your labour companion to help you. If you're really tired, lie down on your left-hand side and let your companion hold your top leg while you are pushing.

CROWNING

When it is time for your baby's head to be born, your midwife will advise you to pant rather than push with your contractions. Try a combination of panting and blowing while thinking to yourself:

'I will not push'
(pant / pant / pant / blow).

This will help your perineum to stretch gently so that you don't tear and your baby's head is not forced into the world in a manner that will probably leave him with a headache for a long time! The pushing stage may take a great deal

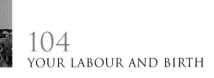

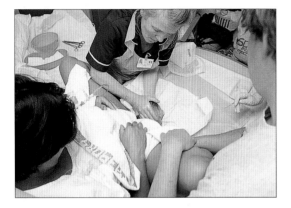

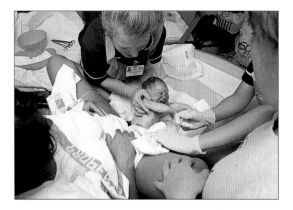

Some women fall instantly in love with their babies. And some don't. They grow to love them over a period of days, perhaps months. You have to let go of the fantasy baby of your pregnancy and adjust to the real baby in your

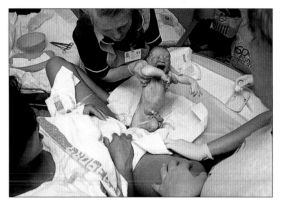

SOME BIRTH EXPERIENCES

'It had been a long labour and I was exhausted, but I had a tremendous feeling of achievement afterwards – I had succeeded in giving birth.'

'I wasn't remotely interested in the baby. I just wanted – more strongly than I've ever wanted anything – to be left alone. In peace.'

'I certainly didn't feel an overwhelming sense of love for him.'

'I just couldn't believe that I'd got a baby and that everything was OK.'

'I looked at her and knew I would do anything for her for the rest of my life.'

arms. This new little person will inevitably be different from the one you imagined and getting to know him properly takes time.

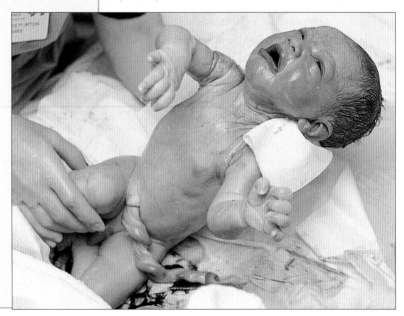

INTO YOUR ARMS

Touch is your new baby's most highly developed sense. What she most needs in the first hours of her life is to *feel* you close to her. Unwrap the blankets so that she can touch your skin. Keep bright lights away from her – her eyes must be dazzled by the rapid change from the darkness of the uterus to the brilliance of her new surroundings. Her ears are still full of amniotic fluid so she is protected from the loud noises around her, but she will still be able to hear your voice and will recognise it as the same voice that she heard in the womb for many months past.

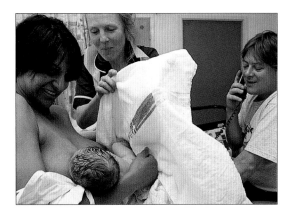

Don't be afraid to take your baby into bed with you; most hospitals allow this now and curling up with your new baby is surely the nicest way to spend the first hours of her life.

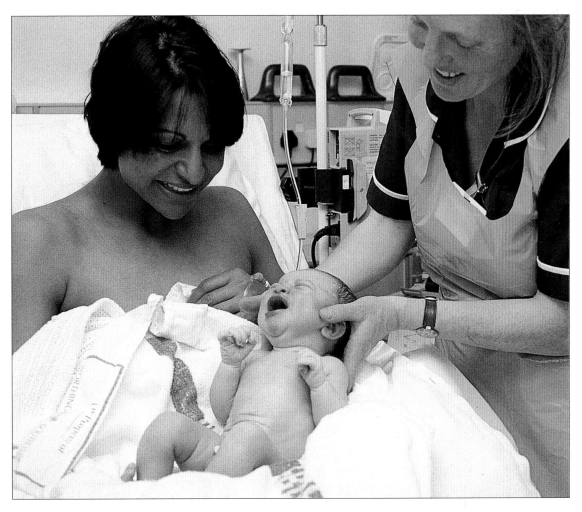

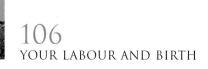

ASSISTED DELIVERIES

Sometimes when the second stage of labour, the pushing stage, is very long and the baby's heartbeat begins to show signs that he is under stress, a helping hand may be needed.

The most usual reasons for a slow second stage are:

• Weak contractions because the mother is exhausted.

• The pelvic floor has relaxed so the baby may not have turned into the best position for birth.

• The mother may not feel the urge to push because she has had an epidural.

FORCEPS OR VENTOUSE?

Under such circumstances, forceps or ventouse (suction) might be suggested to help the baby be born. The pros and cons of each method are summarised in the box below:

When you see your midwife for your next antenatal appointment, ask her to give you some information about assisted deliveries at the hospital where you will be going:

• Is ventouse available?

• What percentage of assisted deliveries are forceps, and what percentage ventouse?

• Are the doctors trained in ventouse delivery?

• Are any midwives trained in ventouse delivery?

• Are there circumstances in which it would not be possible to choose between forceps and ventouse?

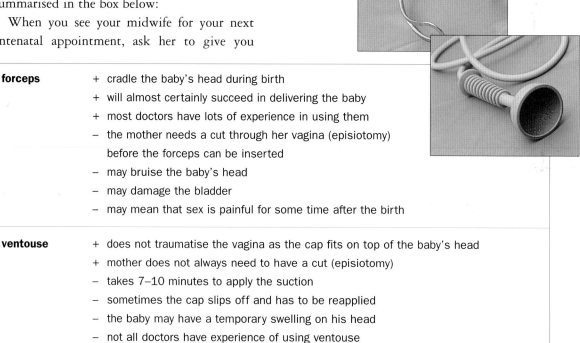

forceps	+ cradle the baby's head during birth
	+ will almost certainly succeed in delivering the baby
	+ most doctors have lots of experience in using them
	– the mother needs a cut through her vagina (episiotomy) before the forceps can be inserted
	– may bruise the baby's head
	– may damage the bladder
	– may mean that sex is painful for some time after the birth
ventouse	+ does not traumatise the vagina as the cap fits on top of the baby's head
	+ mother does not always need to have a cut (episiotomy)
	– takes 7–10 minutes to apply the suction
	– sometimes the cap slips off and has to be reapplied
	– the baby may have a temporary swelling on his head
	– not all doctors have experience of using ventouse

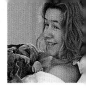

HAVING AN ASSISTED DELIVERY

For an assisted delivery, you will be asked to lie on the bed and probably, to put your legs up in stirrups. A paediatrician (doctor specialising in care of babies and children) will be called so that your baby can be examined as soon as he is born. If you do not already have an epidural in place, you will be offered either pudendal block analgesia to ensure that you feel nothing while the delivery is taking place, or a local anaesthetic delivered to the perineum.

The forceps come in two parts and the doctor places the first one gently round your baby's head and then positions the second on the other side. There is a mechanism to secure the blades (the name for the cupped part of the forceps) so that they are in no danger of slipping. The doctor will then ask you to push when you have a contraction and she will pull at the same time to bring your baby into the world.

If you choose ventouse, you may not need to be cut. The cup will be placed on your baby's head like a skull cap. Suction is gradually applied to remove the air from the cup and

STITCHES AND HOW TO COPE

While you are being stitched:
- say if you can feel anything – stitching should be a painless procedure
- cuddle your baby
- try to relax

Afterwards:
- keep your stitches clean and dry
- eat plenty of fibre (cereal, vegetables, fruit with the skin on) so you don't need to strain to have your bowels open
- drink plenty and wee regularly
- try arnica tablets to ease the bruising (available from most chemists)
- tell your midwife if you have severe pain or any mucky discharge from your stitches
- putting salt in your bath water does not help your stitches heal, but a warm bath is very relaxing and many women find a salt bath very soothing.

make it adhere to your baby's head. As with forceps, the doctor then pulls as you push and together, you deliver your baby.

With either forceps or ventouse, your baby may look a little odd when he is born. There can be bruising or swelling and the head may not be quite symmetrical. Within a few days, the bruising will fade and the swelling disappear.

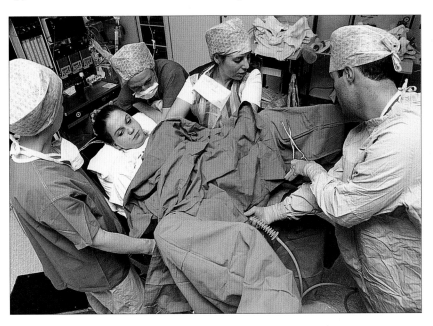

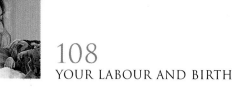

CAESAREAN BIRTH

About one in six women now has a caesarean birth, and up to half of all those caesareans are unplanned. Read this section anyway, so that you will be a little bit prepared.

There are two types of caesarean. With an *emergency* caesarean, an on-the-spot decision is made to perform a caesarean because the condition of your baby has suddenly deteriorated either during pregnancy or labour.

With an *elective* caesarean, factors affecting either your health or your baby's or both, and that you and your professional carers have known about for some time, lead to the decision to book you in for a caesarean.

An emergency caesarean tends to be a fairly high-stress scenario; things happen very quickly. You and your birth companion may feel frightened and out of control, although the best hospitals always find time, even in an emergency situation, to keep you informed. With an elective caesarean, the atmosphere is much calmer. You have probably known for some time the date on which your baby is to be born; all your preparations are made and you have had the chance to talk to your midwife and obstetrician about what will happen.

BEFORE THE OPERATION

A number of procedures take place immediately before a caesarean:
- You sign a consent form.
- You take off all your jewellery; if you have a wedding ring which you don't want to remove, your midwife will cover it with tape.
- You take out your contact lenses.
- You are asked to shave the top centimetre of your pubic hair (or your midwife will do this).
- You are given a small quantity of liquid to drink to neutralise any acid in your stomach.
- An anaesthetist puts a drip into your arm.
- He or she then gives you a spinal injection or an epidural.
- Monitors are placed on your chest to trace your heartbeat.
- A midwife puts a catheter (small tube) into your bladder.
- Your position on the operating table is adjusted so that you are tipped slightly onto your left-hand side.

It is rare nowadays for caesareans to be performed under general anaesthetic. You lose less blood and recover more quickly if you have a spinal or epidural and stay awake during the operation. You can also see and probably hold your baby as soon as she is born. Only in the event of an acute emergency, in order to

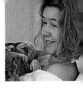

achieve the speediest possible delivery, is it likely that a caesarean might be carried out under general anaesthetic.

If you know you are going to have a caesarean, and are terrified of being awake, discuss your fears with your obstetrician. You may be able to choose a general anaesthetic.

THE OPERATION

The incision is made low down on your abdomen at the level of your pubic hair. During the operation, you might feel strange 'rummaging' sensations inside you; this is quite normal and doesn't mean your anaesthetic isn't working properly. The sensations are odd, but not painful. Your baby will be born within 10 minutes of the surgeon starting the operation. Providing she is well, you can hold her in your arms while the surgeon sews you up again. This takes about 30 to 40 minutes. The skin layer is closed with single stitches, a running stitch, or perhaps with metal clips or surgical glue.

RECOVERING

How quickly you recover from your caesarean is likely to depend on how well prepared you were beforehand. In this respect, women who have had an elective caesarean tend to fare better. If you have had an emergency caesarean, you will probably have been through a very frightening situation when you thought your baby's life was at risk and perhaps your own. One minute you were in the delivery room and the next in theatre, surrounded by people in green gowns and white masks. You might have felt totally out of control. It takes a while to absorb what has happened and your body needs time to recover, especially if labour had been going on for many hours before the caesarean was decided upon.

CAESAREAN SECTION

A large number of people are likely to be present during a caesarean:

- Surgeon (a consultant obstetrician or senior registrar).
- Assistant surgeon (probably a more junior doctor).
- Theatre nurse.
- Midwife.
- Anaesthetist.
- Swab nurse (whose job is to make sure no swabs are left inside you).
- Paediatrician (specialist children's doctor who will check your baby over when she is born).
- Operating department practitioner (whose job is to maintain the theatre).
- Student midwives, doctors or nurses (if you are happy for them to be there).
- Your birth companion (provided you are having a local and not a general anaesthetic).

Be kind to yourself and don't expect to be up and about as quickly as women who have had uncomplicated vaginal deliveries. In the first few days, make sure that you ask for pain relief whenever your tummy starts to hurt. Ask your partner or friend to bring you some high-waisted knickers that won't press on your scar, and some peppermint cordial that you can dilute with water and drink to help with the wind that gets trapped inside you when you have surgery! Ring the bell for your midwife to pass you your baby whenever you want to hold him.

There needs to be someone at home to look after you for at least a week after your discharge from hospital. You need plenty of rest to make a full recovery. Simply feeding your baby is the only task that you should have to do.

THIRD STAGE OF LABOUR

All through pregnancy, your placenta acted as your baby's support system, bringing oxygen and nourishment, filtering out harmful substances and disposing of waste. Now its job is done.

The third stage of labour is when the placenta or afterbirth comes away from the wall of the uterus, passes quickly down the vagina and is delivered. Provided you have had a normal labour with no interventions (i.e. your labour wasn't induced or speeded up, you didn't have any kind of pain relief except gas and air, and you pushed your baby out into the world yourself) you could choose to have a natural (physiological) third stage.

This means:
• After your baby is born, the midwife does not cut your baby's cord until it has stopped pulsating.
• She waits for your uterus to contract and push the placenta out.
• She doesn't press on your tummy or pull on the cord to help the placenta out.
• The placenta is delivered 10 to 20 minutes after the birth of your baby.

However, in many hospitals, it is routine to carry out a 'managed' third stage, both for mothers who have had a natural birth and for those who have had interventions.

A managed third stage means:
• As your baby's shoulders are being born, you are given an injection into your thigh of a drug called syntometrine.
• The midwife clamps and cuts the cord as soon as your baby is born.
• She watches the cord carefully and when she sees it lengthen she knows that the placenta has come off the wall of the uterus.

• She then grasps the cord and draws the placenta out of the vagina.
• The placenta is delivered within 7 minutes of you giving birth.

MANAGED OR UNMANAGED?

There is a great deal of argument amongst health professionals about whether a natural or a managed third stage is preferable, but there is no doubt that it is *not* a good idea to mix the two procedures.

If you are having a natural third stage, there must be no interference at all with the cord, and your body must do all the work of expelling the placenta itself. If you are having a managed third stage, your midwife must actively deliver the placenta.

There's also no doubt that if you have had any kind of intervention in your labour, a managed third stage would be safer for you. It helps protect you against haemorrhage and, while your baby is deprived of some blood that would have passed to him had the cord been allowed to pulsate until it naturally stopped, this does not seem to affect healthy, term babies.

THE PLACENTA

Have a look at the placenta before the midwife takes it away to examine it in the sluice. This is the amazing organ that has looked after your baby for nine months, providing her with all

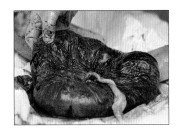
the oxygen and nutrients she needed to grow and thrive, taking away all her waste products, and producing the hormones that maintained your pregnancy. The word 'placenta' means 'flat cake' in Greek because it was believed that babies ate this cake in the womb.

It is deep red on one side, rather like liver, greyish on the other and divided into many lobes. The cord is usually attached in the middle. You will also be able to see the membranes that contained your baby and the amniotic fluid or waters that she was floating in.

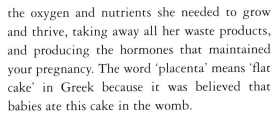

The placenta belongs to you. If you want to take it home, bury it in the garden and plant a tree over it in memory of the birth of your child, you can do so. If you don't want to, the hospital will dispose of it safely.

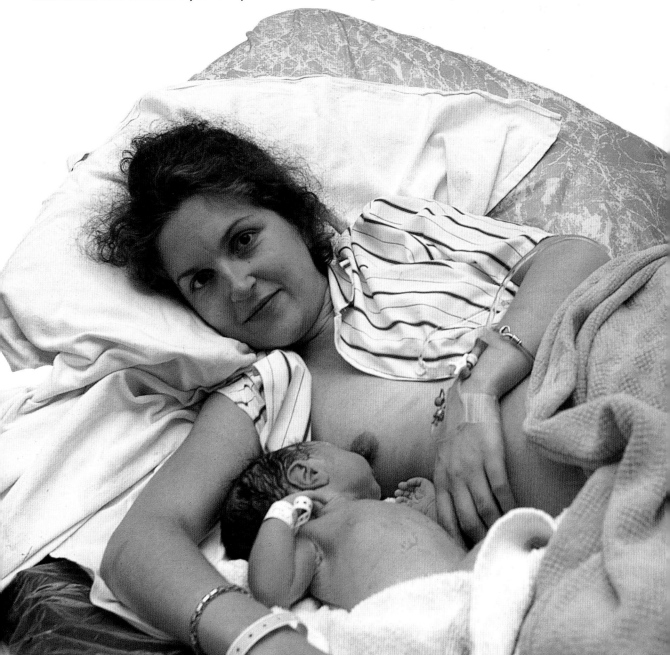

YOU AND YOUR NEW BABY

At last you have your baby in your arms and can spend as much time as you want getting to know him. Although he is now a separate being, there is still a deep connection – your baby can't survive without you.

Soon after delivery, your baby will be checked over by your midwife. A few days later a slightly more detailed examination will be performed by a paediatrician (children's doctor). If you had your baby at home, your GP will visit to carry out this check.

Your baby will probably be examined lying in her cot or on your bed. You should have a clear view and there should be plenty of time for the doctor to explain what she is doing and answer your questions. (See the panel on page 115 'Baby health checks'.)

THE CORD

Your baby's umbilical cord is literally her lifeline throughout pregnancy. Within minutes of her birth, it is clamped with forceps and cut, thus separating her from her placenta.

A short time later, a small, white plastic clamp is snapped in place over the stump of cord left protruding from her belly button. This clamp is there to make sure that no blood is lost from the cord. Your midwife will remove this clamp when your baby is three days old, and the risk of bleeding is past.

The technique for cleaning the cord stump varies from hospital to hospital. You will probably be told simply to wipe the stump with clean water and dry with a cotton wool ball each time you change your baby's nappy. Some hospitals may ask you to sprinkle on a little antiseptic powder.

Try and keep the cord stump and clamp outside your baby's nappy. (You may have to fold the top of the nappy over to do this.) This will stop the stump getting wet with urine – especially if you have a baby boy.

The short length of cord left will dry and shrivel over the next few days until it detaches when your baby is about a week old. There may be one or two specks of blood when this happens

Getting to know each other
– call it playing, call it love.
You're his first relationship.

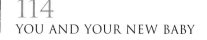
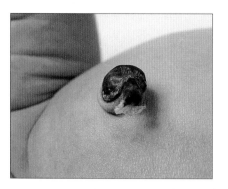

but this will not hurt your baby. She will then be left with a normal looking navel.

Continue to keep the cord clean until it falls off. Do tell your midwife if your baby's cord stump bleeds, looks sticky or has an unpleasant smell. These may be signs of infection.

YOUR BABY'S NAPPIES

Your baby will have been passing urine for several months while in your uterus. She will have her first wee in the outside world within 24 hours or so of birth. If her nappies are still dry after this time, don't panic. It may simply mean that she passed urine during delivery and it was missed in the general excitement. She will probably not pass much urine at all during the first few days.

During the first days your baby will pass 'meconium' – a thick, greenish-black, tarry substance containing mucus, skin cells, swallowed amniotic fluid, and various digestive products.

Meconium can be very messy! It may be a good idea to apply plenty of barrier cream to your baby's bottom when she is first washed or bathed after delivery. This will make it easier to wipe her skin clean after each bowel motion.

During the first week, provided your baby has started to feed, meconium will gradually become greenish-brown in colour. Midwives call this a 'changing stool'. It's a useful sign that your baby is beginning to feed well.

Towards the end of week one, if breastfeeding is going well, your baby's bowel motions will now be very soft and bright yellow in colour. They will have a sweetish, rather pleasant smell. Once you are producing mature milk, your breastfed baby will probably pass 4–5 motions a day. (Over the next few weeks, the frequency of bowel motions may well decrease. She may pass just one bowel motion a day – or one every 2–3 days. This is because there are few waste products from breast milk.)

The bowel motions of a bottle-fed baby are

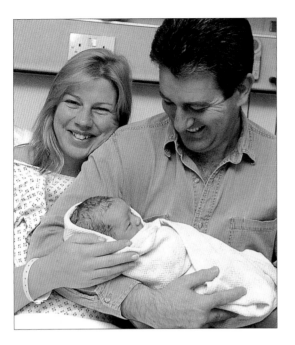

more solid and pale yellowish-brown in colour. They smell rather unpleasant, and are passed more regularly than those of a breastfed baby.

Soft, yellow bowel motions and 6–7 wet nappies in 24 hours, are welcome signs that your breastfed baby is getting plenty of milk. A bottle-fed baby may have fewer bowel motions, but should also have 6–7 wet nappies a day.

Very frequent, greenish bowel motions (after the first five days) and an unsettled baby, may be a sign that your breastfed baby is not getting a balanced breastfeed. This may happen if she is not well latched on to the breast during feeding, or is being taken off the breast before she has had a proper feed.

Very infrequent bowel motions, few wet nappies, and dark, scanty urine may be signs that your baby (breast or bottle-fed) is not getting enough to eat. (It may sometimes be hard to tell whether or not your baby has had a wee, because a disposable nappy may absorb the urine without trace. You will soon learn to tell whether or not a nappy is wet by the weight of it in your hand.)

BABY HEALTH CHECKS

Soon after birth, a paediatrician or GP will check your baby. She will:

- Observe your baby for general signs of health.
- Check for abnormalities.
- Listen to heart and lungs to ensure all is well.
- Feel her tummy and check her external genitalia (sex organs).
- Watch her movements and check her reflexes.
- Check for congenital dislocation of the hips by gently moving her hip joints.
- Ask you about feeding and your baby's behaviour.
- Ask you if you have any worries or questions.

When your baby is 6–10 days old, your midwife will offer to do a blood test to screen for various metabolic disorders. If you agree to this test, the midwife will take a small sample of blood from your baby. This will then be sent to a specialist laboratory for testing.

Your midwife will tell you what conditions are screened for in your area. Usually, the following are included:

- phenylketonuria
- congenital hypothyroidism
  (Left untreated, these two conditions may lead to mental retardation and other problems. Early diagnosis prevents future handicap.)
- cystic fibrosis
- (in some areas) hereditary blood conditions

The results of the test will be sent to your health visitor and GP within a few weeks. Some hospitals offer infant hearing tests. Your baby will be placed in a special cot, wearing a set of headphones through which various sounds are played. A computer analyses your baby's responses and thus detects any hearing loss. Experts agree that early diagnosis and treatment of deafness play a big part in minimising the problem.

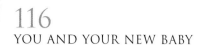

YOUR BODY AFTER THE BIRTH

Although all eyes may now be focused on your baby, it is important that you allow a little time to think about your own health and wellbeing. You're needed more than ever now.

After weeks of waiting, planning, worrying and dreaming, you finally have your baby in your arms. The birth was probably the hardest thing you've ever done, but very special.

Within minutes of the birth of your baby and delivery of your placenta, your uterus shrinks from a bag capable of holding four and a half litres, to a grapefruit-sized pouch of tight muscle. Squeezed tight in the middle of this muscle is the open wound left by your placenta. Already bleeding from this wound has stopped and the area is beginning to heal itself.

Meanwhile, the soft lining of your uterus is being washed away in your lochia (vaginal loss) and a new lining is being built up. The powerful uterine muscles are beginning to shrink; in six short weeks the weight of the empty uterus will reduce from 1,000g to just 60g. This process is called 'involution'.

You will probably find yourself passing large amounts of urine in the first few days as you lose the 2–8 litres of extra fluid carried during pregnancy. At the same time, your heart, lungs and circulation will be returning to normal.

As your placenta leaves your body, its long job finally completed, levels of pregnancy hormones fall rapidly. Smooth muscle tone throughout your body improves quickly – heartburn gets better, constipation is relieved and varicose veins improve. (Unfortunately it takes a bit longer for the effects of hormones on your joints to be reversed; backache and the risk of injury remain potential problems for several months.)

DAILY CHECKS

Each day in hospital, and during each home visit subsequently, your midwife may check:
- temperature and pulse
- blood pressure
- lochia (see box opposite) and the height of your uterus
- legs – to check for signs of thrombosis. Tell your midwife immediately if there's any pain, swelling or redness in your legs
- breasts – for nipple soreness or breast pain, or other signs of feeding difficulties
- perineum – to monitor the healing of any trauma. At the same time, she will probably ask about passing urine or having your bowels open
- how you are feeling generally. Do use this time to ask questions or talk about worries.

YOUR BREASTS

As pregnancy hormones fall, so levels of prolactin rise. Prolactin is the main hormone responsible for milk production. Whether or not you choose to breastfeed, your breasts will

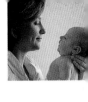
begin to make mature milk to replace the colostrum present throughout most of pregnancy. If you are breastfeeding, feeding your baby in response to her needs will ensure continued production.

If you choose not to breastfeed:

• wear a firm (but not over-tight) bra, night and day, until your breasts return to normal

• if your breasts get very hard, express off a small amount of milk with a little breast pump (don't worry – this will not cause you to make even more milk)

• drink fluids as normal – cutting down may be harmful

• if you feel very uncomfortable, ask your midwife for pain-relieving tablets.

STITCHES

Your perineum is the area between your vagina and your anus. It is this strong wedge of muscle that has to stretch and flatten as the baby's head descends to be born. After the birth, there will be some soreness 'down there' as well as bruising and swelling. (See panel overleaf for how to treat this.)

Sometimes there may be a tear in the perineum or the midwife has to make a small cut (episiotomy) to enlarge the opening for your baby's head. This will be sutured (stitched) by your midwife or doctor. Large tears will also be sutured, to stop bleeding and promote healing, but nowadays smaller tears may or may not be sutured. Many midwives and mothers feel that small tears actually heal better – and are less painful – without stitches. The edges of the wound naturally come together when the legs are closed and, provided there is no infection, generally heal well. (For this to work, though, it's important that you try to keep your legs together as much as possible.) Other people feel that stitches enhance healing.

BLOOD LOSS

'Lochia' is the medical word for the normal discharge from the vagina following childbirth. This is what to expect:

Days 1–3: heavy, dark red discharge that may contain fragments of amniotic membrane and large clots (formed as blood pools in the vagina). This is mainly blood from the placental site.

You will probably have to change your pad every time you go to the toilet. Call your midwife urgently if your loss seems to be heavier than this, or if you feel dizzy and weak.

You may also experience uncomfortable 'after pains' for a few moments each time you feed your baby in the first few days. These are caused by a surge of the hormone oxytocin, stimulated by your baby's suckling. Oxytocin is responsible for the 'let down' (release) of your milk. It also causes your uterus to contract, and so speeds up vaginal discharge.

Your midwife will feel your uterus each day to check that it is well contracted, and is involuting normally.

Days 4–10: significantly lighter, brownish discharge. The placental site is beginning to heal so there is less red blood and more serum (the watery part of blood).

Contact your midwife urgently if, at any stage, your discharge:

• becomes suddenly heavier

• is bright red in colour

• contains lumps of tissue

• has a nasty smell.

Days 10–21: much lighter, yellowish or clear discharge. The lochia now mainly consists of leucocytes (white blood cells involved in healing and fighting infection) and cervical mucus. It may end at three weeks, or may continue off-and-on for up to six weeks.

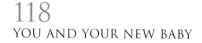

YOUR PERINEUM

Here are some ideas that may help make you more comfortable 'down there' after the birth:

- Keep the area clean. Use a bidet (if there is one) after you've been to the loo, or use a plastic mug or small jug to trickle warm water between your legs as you sit on the toilet. Pat dry with a soft towel.
- Bathe when you can. Some women find a warm bath to which a few drops of lavender oil have been added particularly soothing and relaxing.
- Change maternity pads frequently. Use high-waisted, cotton knickers or disposable briefs.
- Sit on something soft. Many mothers find sitting on a child's swimming ring gives great relief. You may like to consider hiring a 'Valley Cushion' from your local NCT branch.
- Keep moving! It may sound harsh, but walking around as soon as you feel able will help your circulation and reduce swelling.
- You may find pelvic floor exercises impossible to start with, but exercising the pelvic floor does seem to make things more comfortable.
- Consider arnica tablets. It is claimed that arnica reduces bruising and stimulates healing. To be most effective, arnica tablets need to be taken soon after delivery – follow the instructions on the tub or packet carefully. Arnica cream may also be useful but should only be used on intact skin. Witch hazel, calendula or chamomile may also be helpful, applied directly to the skin, and comfrey as a tablet or a tea can help.
- Accept pain relief. Paracetamol, for example, will not interfere with breastfeeding, and will take the edge off perineal pain.
- Chill out! Soak a pad in ice-cold water (or a solution of witch hazel), wring out the excess, and hold it in place against your perineum with another pad. Cold therapies, however, should not be used for longer than one or two days.

AFTER CAESAREAN SECTION

What to expect in the first few days:

- There will be some pain, but it can be controlled. If you had an epidural, this will stay in place for some hours. Or you may be given suppositories which are placed in the back passage and give very good pain relief. Later, you may be offered an analgesic (pain killing) injection. This may be a series of single injections into the muscle of your thigh, or a continuous intravenous infusion of drugs. After two or three days you may find you can manage on a much milder painkiller, like paracetamol.

- You will probably need help to move and to care for your baby. Whether it was a planned or an emergency caesarean section, you have had a major operation. For a few days, you will need help to turn over, sit up, get out of bed, and pick up your baby. It is better to accept a helping hand than strain yourself by struggling alone. Make sure you have a call-bell close to hand, and use it! Your partner or another relative may be able to stay with you to help as well.

- You will have a wound. This will be several inches long, and will probably run across your lower abdomen, just above your pubic hair. It will be covered by a large plaster. Underneath will be either a row of sutures or small metal clips. (Some sutures may be underneath the skin and out of sight. Such sutures do not have to be removed.) When you cough or move it may help to support your wound with your hands (or ask somebody else to do this). Although it will hurt, your wound is very secure. There are sutures not only in the skin, but also through several layers of abdominal and uterine muscles. The skin sutures or clips will be removed after about five days.

- There may be a thin drainage tube leading

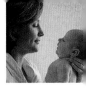
from this wound. This is to remove any blood and fluid and prevent it collecting under the wound. The end of the tube is securely fixed to the wound by a suture, so you cannot accidentally pull it out. There may be thick dark blood in the drainage bottle. This is normal. Your midwife will probably remove the drain after 24–48 hours.

• You will have an intravenous infusion (IVI). This will be dripping fluid directly into your circulation through a fine, flexible tube. You need this extra fluid to make up the blood and fluid loss during surgery, and keep you well hydrated until you are able to drink. Provided you are not feeling sick, you will soon be offered sips of water.

• Your may have a catheter (thin tube) draining your bladder. This will generally be removed within 24–48 hours and you should then be able to pass urine as normal. If you do not have a catheter you may be expected to use a bedpan in bed. Many women find this very difficult. Ask if you can use a commode at the bedside or, better still, be helped to the toilet.

• You will not be able to eat immediately. Following most abdominal operations, it is usual for the gut to take a little while to start working normally again. You may be offered a 'light diet' before gradually starting to eat more normally. During this time, trapped wind may add to your discomfort. Ask your midwife for some peppermint water or other medication. You will know that your gut is working again when you hear the usual gurgling noises.

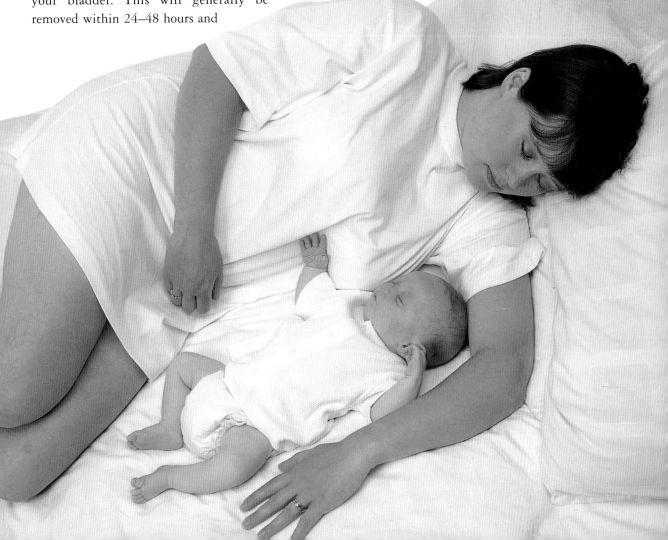

YOUR FEELINGS AFTER BIRTH

Giving birth for the first time is, for most of us, emotionally overwhelming. It's the single most life-changing event of our lives. Small wonder, then, that it can give rise to intense feelings.

The overwhelming relief and thankfulness felt after giving birth is hard to describe to people who have not experienced it. Suddenly, after the intensity of labour, you are floating high with joy, pride, love – you deserve to feel on top of the world. So enjoy this special time. You will remember it for many years to come.

For many women, pregnancy is a very special time, a time when they feel nurtured and unique, on the verge of an exciting adventure. It is normal to feel a sense of regret – even loss – when this time ends. It is natural to mourn the end of something special, even while on the threshold of something even better.

Give yourself time. Tell other people how you feel, but don't be alarmed if they seem not to understand. Talk through the birth with whoever will listen, or write it all down.

DISTRESS

Some women will feel deeper distress.

Maybe the birth was not as you hoped and planned. Perhaps things happened that you didn't want to happen – an assisted delivery or unexpected caesarean section, maybe. Perhaps you feel let down – by your body or by other people. Maybe there were times of great fear and unbearable pain – or perhaps you can't remember much at all. And now all you feel is anger and deep sadness.

Talking about these feelings to others may be very difficult. Your family may not understand:

after all, you have your baby – so do the circumstances of her birth really matter now? Your partner may even be part of the problem, by being absent – in body or spirit – when you needed him. Or he may feel that by telling him of your anger and unhappiness, you are somehow blaming him.

Meanwhile, all around you in hospital other new mothers seem so happy and grateful that you can't help wondering if it's you that is somehow at fault.

If you feel this way, act now. Your distress may fade, but it will probably not go away until it has been faced. Tell your midwife how you feel. Ask her to read through your labour notes, and explain what happened – and why. Better still, ask to speak with the midwife or doctor who cared for you in labour.

You may feel sad for other reasons. Perhaps you are giving birth far from home and family. Maybe the birth of your baby has reawakened your grief for people who have died or gone away, babies you have had before or lost during pregnancy. Maybe the pain and helplessness of labour has brought back deeply unhappy memories from your past.

If you cannot talk things through with somebody in hospital, try to confide in somebody once you are home – your community midwife, maybe, GP, health visitor or antenatal teacher. Perhaps you would find it easier to talk to a stranger – the Birth Crisis Network, maybe, or the Samaritans (see Resources, page

186). Don't dismiss your feelings as unimportant. After all, if your back were hurting as your feelings are hurting, you would seek help – wouldn't you?

AND BABY MAKES THREE...

The early days can be hard for partners, too. They may also be affected by difficulties during labour, and overwhelmed by the enormity of change. They may feel sidelined by events, patronised by health professionals, left out of the closeness developing between you and your baby, useful only for household chores and fetching and carrying.

Overwhelmed by your baby and her needs, worn down by tiredness, inundated with visitors, you may feel that your partner has become yet another responsibility. What you had hoped to be a time of shared happiness, becomes a time of increasing distance and tension. And there just doesn't seem to be the time or the opportunity to sort it out.

Acknowledge these feelings. Tell him that you're having a difficult time – and you know that he is too. Clear the air with a row, make a joke of it, write a loving note – whatever suits your relationship. But you don't need to shoulder the burden of his feelings.

HARD TO LOVE

You may not feel instant and overwhelming love for your baby. Some women don't. Maybe she isn't how you expected, maybe she has turned out to be 'he'. Perhaps she cries a lot, or is ill, or weak – or has another physical problem.

Take each day as it comes. Keep your baby close to you. Hold her skin-to-skin. Feed her, care for her, and sleep with her. Act out love. It may take several weeks, but gradually it will become a reality.

THE 'BABY BLUES'

Midwives reckon that 50–80% of all new mothers suffer the 'baby blues' – a period of weepiness and irritability that sets in around the third to fifth day after birth.

It may be caused by the sudden fall in progesterone following birth. It may also coincide with your milk 'coming in', your baby becoming more unsettled, and your return home from hospital.

Women who give birth at home are much less likely to experience the so-called blues than women cared for in hospital. Several experts have concluded that the 'blues' may be caused, or at least made worse, by such factors as:

- separation from home and family
- impatient and unsympathetic staff
- poor communications and conflict between the mother and those caring for her.

Other experts say that the 'blues' tend to be worse among first-time mothers – especially those with little experience of babies.

The rapid fall in pregnancy hormones may well cause a temporary dip in your mood while your body makes adjustments. But don't let your feelings be dismissed for too long as 'just the baby blues'.

New mothers need sound professional guidance, practical help and loving support. Make sure you're getting your share.

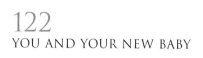

POSTNATAL EXERCISES

You'll recover from the birth more quickly if you can exercise your muscles and joints a little now. It's important to guard your back after the birth, too, and move carefully when bending or lifting.

Continue your pelvic floor exercises (see page 37). If you have had stitches from a tear or episiotomy you will be sore, but the exercise will help improve the circulation and aid healing. Even if you had a caesarean birth, you'll still need to do pelvic floor exercises to prevent problems arising from the effects of pregnancy.

WARNING

Never lie flat on your back and lift both legs in the air. This can do damage when you've just had a baby and your muscles are still weak.

Never lie flat on your back and do sit ups with your feet held down. This will damage your back if your abdominal muscles are weak.

TUMMY STRENGTHENERS

You can start to strengthen abdominal muscles again now, as you did in pregnancy (see the antenatal exercises on page 34).

Get onto all fours and do this exercise with your baby. Strengthen the abdominals by pulling your tummy button in towards your spine without moving your back or tilting your pelvis.

At any time during the day, sitting or standing, you can strengthen your abdominal muscles simply by drawing in your tummy button in this way.

As the weeks pass and your abdominal muscles get stronger, you can try adding a leg lift to strengthen your back muscles. Make sure you keep the leg level with your back and avoid arching your back or lifting your head up. Repeat the lift 6 to 8 times each leg.

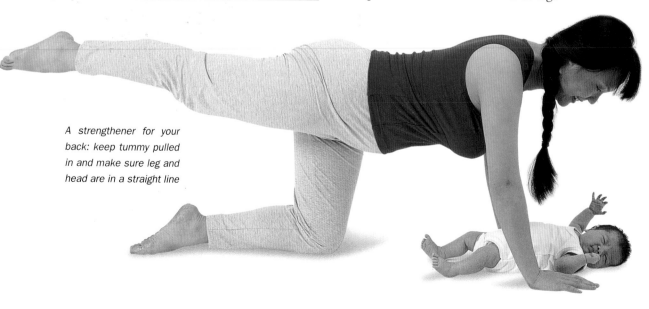

A strengthener for your back: keep tummy pulled in and make sure leg and head are in a straight line

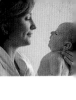

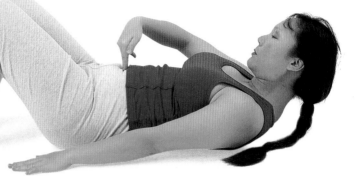

REC CHECK

The 'rectus abdominis' is a major muscle that travels the length of your front. The right and left halves have to separate during pregnancy, to make room for your growing bump. Before you start doing any sit ups, it's important to check whether these two halves are coming together again.

You can do this with a 'rec check'. Lie on your back with your knees bent and place three fingers of your right hand just below your belly button. Slide your left hand down the floor towards your feet and lift your head and shoulders off the bed or floor. As you lift up you should feel two hard ridges of muscle on either side of your right hand. This should tell you how well your abdominal muscles are coming together. As you exercise and your muscles get stronger, the gap between the two ridges of muscle should narrow until it is about the width of a fingertip.

CURL UPS

If the gap is more than three finger-widths apart, then only do gentle curl ups with both hands crossed over your abdomen, as shown.

Keeping your abdomen flat with your hands, gently lift your head and shoulders off the floor to strengthen the straight abdominal muscles and then slowly lower. Keep the angle between your chin and your chest the same throughout the exercise and keep breathing – 'out' as you lift and 'in' as you lower. Do this exercise 6 to 8 times.

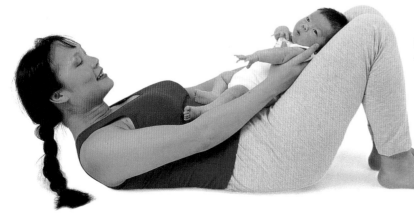

CURL UPS WITH A BABY

As the gap in the rectus muscle narrows and you get stronger, you can do the same curl ups with your baby lying against your thighs.

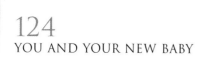

THE EARLY DAYS AT HOME

The big moment has come: taking your baby home from hospital!
You may be surprised by how mixed-up you feel. There'll be
excitement, and pride, certainly, but also some anxiety.

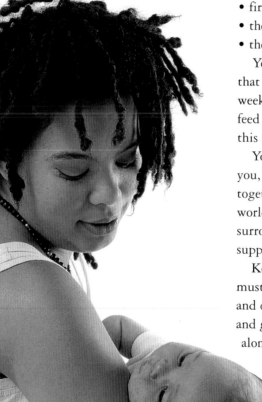

Some women find it quite hard to leave hospital with their new baby, especially if they have been an in-patient for some time. After all, in hospital there are no domestic worries, help is always on hand, there's a reassuring routine to the days – and now, suddenly, you feel like you're out on your own! It can be quite scary.

These are your priorities:
• first your baby
• then yourself
• then everyone else.

Your baby needs food, comfort and love. It's that simple. Accept that, for the next few weeks, your absolute priority is learning how to feed your baby. Nothing is more important at this stage.

You may find it helps to take a 'babymoon' – you, your baby and your partner at home together, preferably in bed, with the rest of the world kept firmly at bay. Or you may prefer to surround yourself with women friends and supporters.

Keep your baby close to you. Think what it must be like for her: one moment she is curled and cosy in your womb, surrounded by warmth and gentle sounds – the next she is exposed and alone. Hold and carry your baby as much as you physically can. The closer she is to you, the quicker your response to her needs. You will be teaching her about security, love and warmth.

Within a few short hours, you will be the expert regarding your baby: you will know more about her, her needs and how to meet them than any midwife or doctor in the world. You will learn that she likes to be wrapped firmly in her shawl, that she likes her head to be stroked – but she hates her bottom being washed. You may take ages doing things and feel incredibly clumsy – but so what? You're the only mother she's ever known and, as far as she is concerned, you are perfect!

You, too, need food, comfort and love. You may be tempted to put everyone else's needs in front of your own, but if you are not well-fed, rested and happy, your baby will soon feel the effects. So:

• Make eating a priority. Write a list of your favourite snacks and pin it up in the kitchen. Then other people can quickly prepare the food you want without a lot of questions.

• When your baby is asleep, or settled with somebody else, do something you enjoy.

• Be ruthless with visitors. Tell them you need to rest. Wearing nightclothes for the first few days at home will reinforce this message.

MOTHERING THE MOTHER

In many traditional societies, new mothers are segregated, cared for and nurtured for several weeks – expected to do little else except feed their babies and rest.

Plan ahead. Who is going to mother you when your baby is born? Who will cook, clean, shop, wash, fetch and carry, hold your baby while you bath, shield you from visitors, make endless cups of tea, mop your tears, accept your grumbles, tell you you're great – yet expect very little in return? Is this really a one-man job?

KEEPING YOUR BABY CLOSE

Simply by holding your baby you will be meeting her need for security and love. She will cry less and settle quicker. And the longer you hold her, the more you will want to do so.

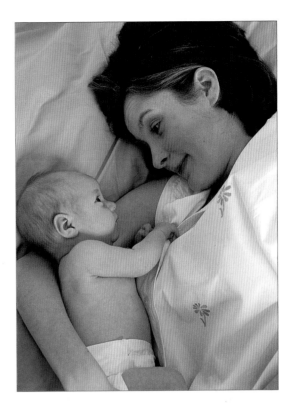

This is not 'spoiling' your baby. This is helping her make the transition from the womb to the outside world. The early security of your presence will make the inevitable separations to come the easier for her to bear.

Improvise your own baby carrier. Use 2m of thin cotton fabric. Tie the two ends in a loose reef knot, and put your head and one arm through the loop of fabric. Adjust the knot so that the fold of the fabric is slightly above waist level, and tighten. Lie your baby in the fold and pull up a layer of fabric between her body and your chest. Tuck the sides of the fabric in under her head and feet, so she is held snugly in a hammock of fabric. Support her with one hand, if you wish, but let the fabric take her weight.

Invest in a commercial baby carrying sling. These are shaped and worn in much the same way as the home-made sling. Most have some sort of buckle to enable quick adjustment, and the edges and neck strap are padded.

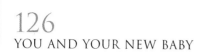
YOU AND YOUR MIDWIFE

Your midwife will probably visit you every day until your baby is 10 days old. In some areas, your midwife may offer her support for up to 28 days. In both cases, you will probably meet your health visitor when your baby is about 2 weeks old.

Few other countries in the world have this system of home midwifery care. We are very lucky.

Although your midwife will try to tell you when she is likely to visit you each day, these arrangements may end up being very vague. She may be delayed in an antenatal clinic, responding to an emergency, or stuck in traffic. This can be irritating and inconvenient for everybody, not least your midwife. There is no easy answer, except patience.

You may find that your midwife offers 'selective' visits. This means that she may not necessarily call every day. Some experienced mothers prefer this system. In theory, it frees the midwife to spend more time with inexperienced or unsupported mothers.

On the other hand, selective visiting can leave some mothers feeling insecure and anxious. Although your midwife will involve you in deciding when she should visit, you may find it hard to say what you really want. It's easy

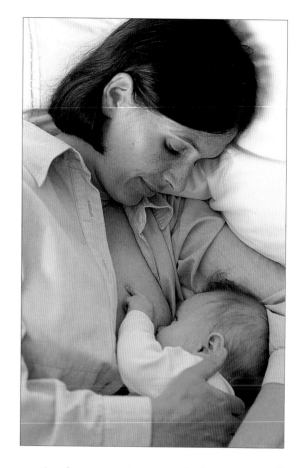

to simply agree when somebody says, 'you'll manage without me tomorrow, won't you?'

Make sure you have a contact telephone number for your midwife. Check if this is also the number to use for emergencies – feeding problems or health concerns 'after hours'.

Jot down worries and questions when you think of them during the day (or night), ready for your midwife's visit.

If you feel you need a different pattern of visits from the one offered, do say so. Many mothers need extra help to get breastfeeding established, for example.

SLEEPING TOGETHER

Your baby is content, you sleep better, breastfeeding is easier, bottle-feeding is cosier – and it feels good! So why not give it a try?

'I'll roll over and squash her.' No you won't – unless, maybe, you've taken sleeping tablets or had too much alcohol to drink.

'She'll get too hot.' Video recordings of mothers sleeping with their babies show how they frequently touch their babies to check their temperature, and adjust the bedding accordingly. She won't need to wear much – just a nappy and vest. Alternatively, some mothers prefer to have their babies resting on top of the bedclothes, under a baby blanket – rather than beneath the adult duvet.

'I need my own space.' Fair enough. How about some sort of compromise – your baby's cot beside your bed maybe, so you can easily move her close to feed her?

REDUCING THE RISK OF COT DEATH

Protect your baby from smoke. Be aware that one piece of research has shown that if you smoke, your baby may be at increased risk of 'cot death' if she sleeps with you, either in bed at night or on a sofa during the day. This is because even when asleep, smokers breathe out harmful chemicals.

Consider breastfeeding. Most experts now agree that breastfed babies are less likely than formula-fed babies to become victims of cot death. This may be because breast milk offers protection against infection and illnesses – or could be because of other advantages conferred by breastfeeding that we don't yet fully understand.

Prevent over-heating. Babies naturally lose heat through their heads, so if you cover her head while indoors she may get too hot. If she is sleeping in a cot, lie her with her feet to the foot of the cot, so she cannot wriggle down under the bedclothes. Do not use a duvet (it may ride up over her head) or cot 'bumpers' (these may make her too hot). Feel her tummy to assess her temperature, and dress her accordingly.

Be alert for signs of illness and contact your GP, midwife or health visitor quickly.

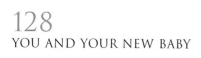
BREAST OR BOTTLE?

Deciding how you will feed your baby is probably one of the most important decisions to make during pregnancy. Consider the options and make the choice that's right for you.

Breastfeeding is best for babies and for women, and breastfeeding without any formula milk or solid food for six months is the 'gold standard' of feeding to aim for.

Your breasts have been preparing for feeding for the last nine months: tingling and heaviness of the breasts is one of the very first symptoms of pregnancy, the milk-producing areas of the breast start enlarging and your nipples gradually grow more prominent. From as early as four months, colostrum (a form of early milk) is present.

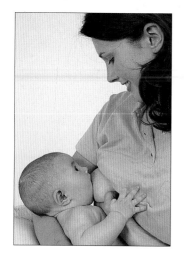

You may find it helpful to think of the feeding decision not in terms of 'how' to feed your baby, but 'what' to feed her. In other words, you are not just considering a choice between breast and bottle, but between breast milk and formula milk. And whereas formula milk can only be given in a bottle, breast milk can be given directly from the breast or in a bottle.

If you chose to breastfeed you can (once your supply is established) combine breastfeeding and feeding with formula milk in a way that suits your personal circumstances. Your baby will still receive many of the advantages of breast milk.

If you choose to bottle-feed your baby from the very beginning, it can be very hard to change to breastfeeding. If you are undecided, it's therefore best to start breastfeeding. Your baby will benefit enormously from even a few feeds of colostrum. Colostrum is rich in antibodies and other substances that protect against illness and infection.

WHY BREAST IS BEST

There are many proven health advantages to breast milk. Research has shown that premature babies who are given breast milk have higher IQs and a much lower risk of necrotising enterocolitis (a potentially fatal bowel disorder).

Scientific research has also proved that babies who are fully breastfed for three to four months are less likely to get:
- severe diarrhoea
- a chest infection that needs to be treated in hospital
- middle-ear infections
- urine infections
- eczema or chest wheeze if their family has a history of allergies
- diabetes as a child.

Breastfeeding also gives protection against numerous other diseases and disorders and the advantages last well into childhood. There are many long-term health advantages for women, too, including some protection against breast cancer. It's certainly true that breast is best.

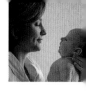

WHAT YOU NEED

- 2–3 nursing bras.
- A pack of 6 washable breast pads.
- Plenty of loose tops to wear.
- Catalogues from mother-and-baby shops.

Even if you do not usually wear a bra, you will probably feel more comfortable doing so while you are breastfeeding. Wait until you are about 36 weeks pregnant before getting yourself measured. Most department stores' lingerie departments offer a measuring service, as do many high street mother-and-baby shops. Many NCT branches have Mava bra agents. You can visit them at home to try on different styles.

A good breastfeeding bra:
- is made of cotton or cotton-rich fabric
- supports your breasts without squashing them flat
- has wide, non-stretchy straps
- does not put pressure on your nipples
- has plenty of hooks-and-eyes to adjust fit
- is easy to open one-handed.

Some women leak a lot of milk in the early weeks of breastfeeding, some not at all. Buy some pads (disposable, if you prefer) but don't open the pack until you are sure you need them.

Loose tops that you can lift up are best for breastfeeding (and more discreet). You won't need much else – nipple shields, maybe, or a small bottle in which to give expressed milk. It's probably best to ask somebody to buy these things if (not when) you need them. Having one or two store catalogues to hand will help you check what is available.

BOTTLE-FEEDING

Today's formula milks have been developed so that they mimic the composition of breast milk as closely as possible. If you choose to bottle-feed,

---

BREASTFEEDING OR BOTTLE-FEEDING?

Although 'breast is best', there are advantages to both the baby feeding methods.

BREASTFEEDING:
- the quality of the milk is nutritionally superior and changes as the baby grows to meet all her needs
- there is less chance of developing allergies
- breast milk contains antibodies that confer distinct health benefits
- breast milk is free, needing only a small amount of extra food from you
- there is no preparation time and no need for sterilisation
- breast milk is specifically made for human babies – it is the best possible food for them, helping development of the brain and nervous systems, and protecting against gastro-intestinal and middle-ear problems.
- research indicates that breastfeeding is also beneficial for mothers, giving some protection against certain forms of cancer and osteoporosis
- breast milk is always delivered at exactly the right temperature.

BOTTLE-FEEDING:
- the responsibility for feeding can be shared more equally between the parents and other carers
- some people think that bottle-fed babies sleep for longer than their breastfed counterparts and there is evidence to support this
- the amount that a baby takes in a feed can be measured
- there is no change of feeding methods if you are returning to work.

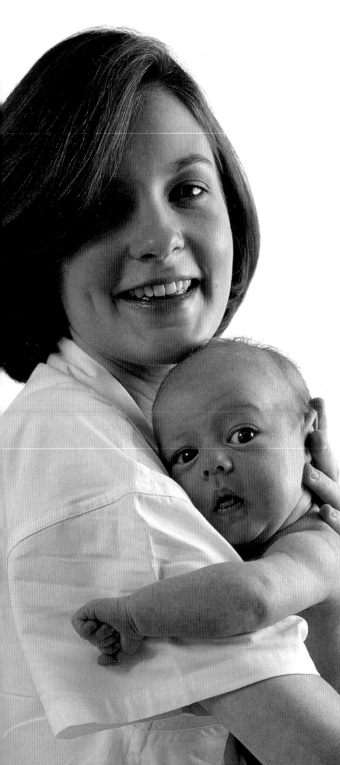

you will need the following equipment:
• powdered milk suitable for newborn babies
• 6 standard size (250ml) feeding bottles, and bottle brush
• 6 'newborn' or 'slow-flow' teats, and covers
• a steam steriliser or other method of sterilising bottles, teats and other equipment
• a large, wide-based jug for hot water in which to gently reheat bottle (or bottle warmer)

Do not use a microwave to heat any kind of baby milk. 'Hot spots' may form and your baby's mouth may be badly burnt.

Choosing formula milk

'Whey-dominant' milks are thought to be best for new babies. Ask your midwife, health visitor or pharmacist for impartial advice on what sort of milk to use.

The range of formula milks available can be quite bewildering. In terms of ingredients there is probably very little to choose between the major brands. Manufacturers are all quick to implement new safety standards and innovative ingredients. Your midwife or health visitor will be able to recommend brands.

Types of formula milk

Almost all of the formula milks sold for babies are based on cows' milk protein. They fall into two groups:
• 'whey-dominant' milks are considered most suitable for newborn babies. Brand names often suggest this – but read the container carefully to be sure
• 'casein-dominant' milks are generally marketed as being suitable for older, 'hungrier' babies – although some experts believe there is no real advantage.

Baby milks are sold in powdered form in tubs or packets. Some milks are also available ready-mixed in small cartons. They tend to be expensive, but may be very useful for days out or travelling.

A few women choose to feed their babies on soya-based baby milk. This decision is usually made because they believe their babies to be allergic to either cows' milk protein or to lactose (milk sugar). The problem is that a significant proportion of these babies will also be allergic to soya protein. Other worries about soya milk include the use of genetically modified crops in their manufacture, and allegedly high levels of harmful chemicals such as phytoestrogens. Do get expert advice before using soya-based milk.

Bottles and teats
Small feeding bottles look attractive, but your baby will soon out-grow them. On the other hand, some mothers find it is useful to have 1–2 smaller bottles for giving drinks of cooled, boiled water between milk feeds. Wide-neck bottles are easier to clean than standard bottles. Some bottles are easier to hold than other bottles – so experiment before buying.

'Newborn' or 'slow-flow' teats have just one hole in the tip, so the flow of milk is controlled and your baby is encouraged to suck vigorously. (Medium-flow, fast-flow, and 'variflow' teats are more suited to older babies.) Make sure the teats fit your chosen bottles.

Choose from latex (natural rubber) or silicon teats:
• latex teats are soft and pliable, but can deteriorate fairly quickly and so may need to be replaced more frequently than silicone teats
• silicone teats are more durable and easier to clean, but may be split if punctured. They are more expensive than latex teats.

Both types of teats should be carefully inspected before and after use. Throw away any teats that are cracked or tacky. Loose pieces may harm your baby, or provide a breeding ground for bacteria.

Teats are available in a variety of designs:
• 'standard' teats are the traditional round-ended shape
• 'orthodontic' teats are shaped to follow the contours of a baby's mouth
• 'anti-colic' teats allow air to enter the bottle during feeding, and so may prevent a vacuum forming. The baby can feed without interruption, and air swallowing is reduced.

COMBINING BREAST AND BOTTLE

More and more women are now choosing mixed feeding, which means using a flexible combination of breast milk and formula milk for their baby. This may be because you are returning to work before you are ready to give up breastfeeding or simply because you and your partner wish to share the feeding.

Your baby will need to become used to the different textures, smells and techniques of sucking that come with breast and bottle. Your success depends partly on the character of your baby and on how relaxed you and your partner are. Don't rush anything, concentrate on building up an abundant milk supply in the early weeks, maybe introducing a bottle once or twice a week (with either expressed milk, water or formula milk). Remember that as soon as you start to introduce a bottle your own milk supply will slow down, which is why it is important to get your milk supply well established first – and this can take up to six weeks.

Once you have a smooth routine established you will find that your milk supply adapts and you will be able to allow that routine to become more flexible as time goes on. If your milk supply seems to drop too much take the time to breastfeed more often, rest when you can and ensure that you are eating and drinking properly. Within a day or so your milk supply will have increased again.

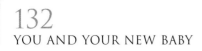

BREASTFEEDING

Breastfeeding is a skill that has to be learned in the days following the birth of your baby – in the midst of recovering from labour and adjusting to the turmoil of new motherhood.

It's a good idea to put your baby to your breast soon after birth. 'Soon' is when your baby and you are ready, whether this is within a few minutes or an hour later. Later, both of you may be tired and sleepy: breastfeeding now means that your baby will have a comforting tummyful of colostrum – and you will know you can do it.

If you give birth in an upright position or sitting in a propped-up position – standing, kneeling or crouching – it will feel natural and easy to reach down and gather your baby in your arms. Take time to look at each other then, when it feels right, hold her against your breast and guide her as she seeks your nipple. Leaning forward slightly will make it easier for her to latch on. You may have given birth lying down or lying on your side. With a normal delivery, the midwife will hand you your baby after the birth once you are comfortable.

Things may take a bit longer if you are lying down following an assisted delivery, with doctors and midwives still attending to you. Don't let this worry you: your baby will also need time to get ready for feeding. In fact, video studies of newborn babies show that, left entirely to their own devices, a baby is happy to spend 60–90 minutes nuzzling and looking for her mother's nipple, before finally latching on to feed. So maybe babies prefer not to be rushed either!

If all is well, your midwife or doctor will place your newborn baby on to your abdomen, covered with a small towel. Support her gently and just enjoy looking at each other. Let her wriggle and move as she wishes. Given time, she may even start inching towards your breasts. Help her if you wish, then let her explore a little more. Eventually she will start 'rooting' (turning towards the nipple and opening her mouth). Now may be the time to either sit up or turn onto your side, so she can latch on to your breast and feed.

GETTING STARTED

First, get yourself comfortable. You will soon find positions that suit you and your baby.

• **Gather together the things you may need** – a drink for you, tissues to mop up dribbles, call-button to summon help, small length of ribbon to tie your clothing clear of your breast, breastfeeding leaflet or guide.

• **Make sure your back is upright, and then think about your back and arm support** – a low, comfortable, upright chair with armrests is ideal – but you probably won't find one in hospital! So make the best of what you have with plenty of firm pillows: under your arms to take the weight of your baby, behind your back to keep you upright, across your lap to lift your baby to breast height. (You won't need all these cushions for ever, but they are useful in the first 4–6 weeks while you and your baby are learning together.)

• **Make sure your lap (hips to knees) is level** to prevent your baby slipping downwards – telephone directories make excellent footstools. If you are breastfeeding in a hospital bed, consider swinging your legs over the side and resting them on the floor or on a low chair. (It's very difficult getting into a good upright position using those sloping metal backrests and a couple of slippery pillows.)

The next step is to get your baby comfortable.

• **Take a few moments to calm her** if she has been crying – talk to her and tell her what is happening. You may find it helps to wrap her securely in a shawl or small blanket for the first few feeds – but make sure she doesn't get too hot. Later, she will probably prefer her hands free to touch and stroke your breast. Undo your bra, and tuck or tie your clothing out of the way.

• **Holding your baby close, turn her whole body towards you, keeping her back and head in a straight line.** Notice how your breast hangs in its natural position and line your baby up so her nose is level with your nipple. (Doing this means that she will have to tilt her head back slightly to reach for your nipple. This gives her room to open her mouth really wide, and get a good latch onto your breast. Imagine how hard it would be for you to eat an apple with your chin tucked down against your chest.)

• **Make sure your baby's head moves freely.** This is very important. As described above, she needs to have room to drop her lower jaw, so she can open her mouth wide to latch on. This is why the 'beginner hold' (as shown in the photograph) is so useful in the early days. Your baby's head is gently supported, rather than held in a fixed

position (as it would be in the crock of your arm). She can open her mouth wider – and you can move her in close to you quickly when she is ready to latch on.

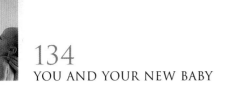
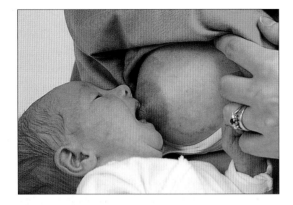

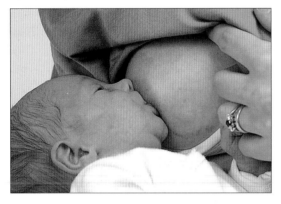

Latch her on

• If you wish, support your breast gently from below, using the flat of your hand. Make sure your fingers are well away from your areola, where they may get in the way as your baby latches on. Be very careful not to press or squeeze the delicate breast tissue: this may cause painful bruising or a blocked milk duct.

• If your baby is not already rooting for the breast, touch her lips with your nipple. Wait for her to open her mouth as wide as a yawn. This may take a few minutes. Remember, her mouth needs to be wide open so she can take in not only your nipple but a good portion of your areola as well. Tell her what you want her to do: 'Open wide. Nice wide mouth. Good girl.' Open your own mouth wide. You may feel daft doing this – but babies imitate facial expressions from a very early age.

• As soon as your baby's jaw drops and her

mouth opens wide, draw her gently but swiftly closer. Make sure her head doesn't curl in as you do this: move her whole body – not just her head. Once she gets a good 'mouthful' of breast, she will draw your nipple further back into her mouth and start suckling.

• It may take several attempts to get this right. Although you may find it very tempting to give in after one or two tries, and just let her get on with it – don't! Your nipples will soon get very, very sore.

A good latch

What it feels like:

• There is no pain. Once you've got going, you should be able to relax (drop those shoulders!), look around, and carry on a normal conversation.

• You are probably aware of a deep, 'drawing' feeling. This may feel very strange to start with, but should not be painful.

• You may notice a tingling, tightening sensation as the oxytocin flows and your milk is 'let down'.

• Although your breasts will fill up between feeds, they will feel comfortable. A good latch ensures that your breasts are effectively 'drained': there will be no hard, painful lumps and no hot, red patches (classic signs of a blocked milk duct and early mastitis).

What 'a good latch' looks like:

• Only a small proportion of your areola is still visible.

• Your baby's chin is firmly in contact with your breast.

• Her nose is clear of your breast, or lightly touching.

• Her mouth is open (as yours would be if you were eating an apple).

• Her cheeks are rounded throughout the feed: she is *suckling* (massaging the breast) not

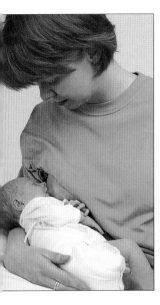

sucking – remember!

• The whole of her lower jaw is moving: you can see muscles working right back near her ears.

If the latch is good, your baby will:

• feed happily at the breast: quickly at first – to stimulate the let down of milk, then more slowly as she enjoys the flow of creamy milk

• stop feeding spontaneously when she has had enough

• be settled afterwards (although she may sometimes want to feed from the other breast soon afterwards).

If breastfeeding hurts

If breastfeeding hurts, something is wrong!

Throughout the first week, the initial few seconds of each breastfeed may be painful. This is because your baby has to draw your nipple to the back of her mouth and, to start with, this may hurt. But, after this few seconds, breastfeeding should not hurt. If it does:

• Ease the tip of your little finger into the corner of your baby's mouth, and move her gently off the breast. Then have another go at latching her on.

• If it still hurts, ask your midwife urgently for help. Ask her to watch you latch your baby on. This will be much more useful than just watching you once you have started.

• Don't be fobbed off! Your nipples will *not* 'harden up' – nor will you 'get used to it'. Ask if there is an infant feeder advisor in the hospital, or another midwife who specialises in breastfeeding support.

If your nipples get sore, blistered or cracked, latching your baby on well is even more important. It may be hard to believe, but even very sore nipples will not hurt during feeding – provided your baby is latched on well. And, once the latch is corrected, nipples heal amazingly quickly.

• Your midwife may suggest you use a dab of cream or a tiny dressing on open sores, to protect them and promote healing.

• Be wary of suggestions to dry your nipples with hair-driers or sunlight! Modern wound management theory suggests that nipple sores and cracks heal best if kept soft and moist.

• If feeding is just too painful to contemplate, your midwife may suggest either resting the sore breast (and expressing off the milk for your baby) – or using a nipple shield. Take time to talk through the pros and cons of both actions before deciding what to do. Whichever method you choose, it should only be necessary for, at the most, 2–3 days.

HOW MUCH, HOW OFTEN?

A generation ago, mothers were encouraged to feed their babies to schedule – according to a timetable. Today, most babies are fed 'on demand' – according to individual need. In other words, the baby is offered the breast whenever she is hungry, and allowed to feed until she has had enough. Some people call this 'baby-led feeding'. (In most countries in the world, it is simply called 'feeding', because it's so obviously the only way to feed a small baby!)

The beauty of this approach lies in its efficiency and convenience. Your breasts produce milk in direct response to how much and how often your baby feeds – so, with baby-led feeding, there is always the right amount of milk waiting for her. Supply matches demand.

You don't have to wait until your baby is

crying before you feed her. Many women find that learning how to breastfeed is much easier if their baby is calm – rather than impatient and upset. You will soon start to notice the signs that your baby is ready to feed – mouth movements, stretching, little noises and so on – and, if in doubt – offer the breast anyway. Your baby will let you know if that is not what she wants!

A baby who is well latched on to the breast will stop feeding when she has had enough: generally after 20–30 minutes, certainly within 40 minutes. (Don't worry – feeds get much quicker as the weeks go by.)

She may want to feed again four hours later – or an hour later. The frequency of feeds will vary a lot throughout the day. (This is not unreasonable: think, for a moment, how often you have a cup of tea, a biscuit, or a glass of water.) Experts reckon that at least eight feeds are needed in every twenty-four hours to ensure good levels of prolactin and adequate milk production. A few babies manage on this number of feeds, but most need a lot more.

If you feel your baby is 'feeding all the time' there are three possibilities:
• she is not latched on well, and so is not getting enough creamy hindmilk to satisfy her (your nipples may also be very sore)
• she is working hard for 12 hours or so to build up your supply of milk (in which case, the frequency of feeds will soon settle now)
• she knows that if she stops suckling, she'll be put into her cot and left all alone – and that's not what she wants at all.

IF YOU GIVE BIRTH BY CAESAREAN

You can still breastfeed, but it may help to be mentally prepared for two possible difficulties:
• In the first few days, you will probably find it difficult to lift and position your baby

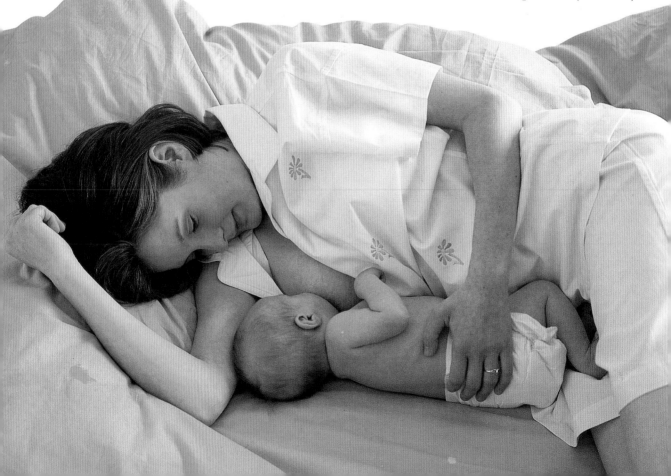

without help, especially if you have a drip in place. It may hurt to hold your baby in the conventional way, across your abdomen.

• If your baby is quite small, a large, soft pillow on your lap may help. Alternatively, you could hold her in the underarm position, body and legs out to one side, supported on a couple of firm pillows. Best of all, try feeding your baby lying down.

• You may find that there is a delay in the changeover between colostrum and mature milk (your milk 'coming in'). This delay seems to be more likely if you have a planned caesarean section, or if you are in labour for only a short time before surgery is needed. This may be because the hormones that play a part during active labour may also help prepare for lactation.

• Feeding your baby frequently in the early days will encourage the production of mature milk. Pay particular attention to getting a good latch, so your baby will get plenty of colostrum.

Feeding lying down

• Get yourself comfortable with 2–3 pillows under your head and, maybe, one behind your back. If you have generous breasts, you will find it helps to have the short end of a pillow under your ribs – so that your lower breast is not squashed against the mattress.

• Lie well over on your side, your lower arm curled under or supporting your head. Your baby should be resting on the mattress in front of you, well over on her side. Support her with your upper arm.

• Line your baby up with your breast. When she roots for the nipple, slide her swiftly on to your breast, in the usual way, making sure that her head is not curled forwards. (You may need somebody to guide you the first few times – you may not be able to see clearly what you are doing!)

GETTING HELP

Midwives and health visitors are specially trained and qualified to advise and support breastfeeding mothers.

• If you need help with breastfeeding, do tell your midwife. Make sure you have a contact telephone number to use for out-of-hours problems. Remember: feeding your baby is vitally important, and feeding difficulties deserve prompt professional attention.

• If you have tried to work with your midwife, but need extra support then contact an NCT breastfeeding counsellor (020 8992 8637) or phone the Breastfeeding Network Supportline (0870 900 8787). There may be other breastfeeding groups active in your area: look out for leaflets and posters in doctors' surgeries and local libraries.

Please remember that breastfeeding counsellors and supporters are all volunteers, with their own family and work commitments. They will do their very best to help you through telephone support and (sometimes) home visits – but may not always be able to give you immediate attention.

• If you cannot get in touch with your midwife and you need urgent help with breastfeeding (especially if you also have worries concerning your baby's health) then telephone the postnatal ward at your local maternity unit for advice.

Above all, don't forget your support network of friends and family who are positive about breastfeeding. Talking about difficulties and frustrations, and sharing ideas and answers will help more than you can imagine. In many societies, new mothers are surrounded and supported by female friends and relatives as they learn to care for and feed their babies. Don't feel you have to struggle on alone.

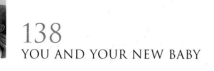
BOTTLE-FEEDING

Feeding your newborn baby should be a special time. Some mothers like to sing and talk to their babies as they are feeding, others prefer to just get to know each other.

Feeds may take quite a while to start with. This is quite normal so don't try and rush things – both of you have a lot to learn.

BOTTLE-FEEDING YOUR BABY

• Try to feed in a calm and restful atmosphere. Take the phone off the hook, and ask not to be disturbed. Quieten your baby if she has been very upset before feeding – if she starts to feed while crying she may take in extra air and get windy.

• Gather together the things you need – bottle of milk warming in a jug of hot water, tissues or bib, drink and snack for yourself.

• Choose a comfortable chair, with good back support. A small footstool or a couple of telephone directories may be useful to raise your knees and level your lap. Pillows under your arms will make it more comfortable to hold your baby for a length of time.

• Some babies like to be swaddled cosily in a shawl for feeding. Others prefer to be able to move their arms, and touch and explore. You'll soon find out what your baby likes. (Take care she doesn't get too hot.)

• Experiment with feeding positions, but make sure her head is always slightly higher than her tummy. You may prefer to hold her tucked in close to your body, with her head resting in the crook of your arm. Or you may like to hold her

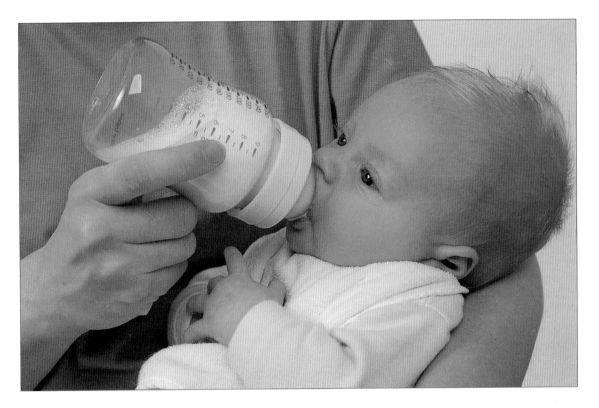

slightly away from you, with her head in your hand and her feet touching your tummy. You both may enjoy the more direct eye contact that is possible in this position. (Some people feel you should alternate the side on which you hold your baby to feed, but this can feel awkward if you are strongly right or left handed.)

• Make sure the milk in the bottle is at a comfortable temperature. Sprinkle a little on the inside of your forearm to test. (Don't heat a bottle of milk in a microwave oven. The milk may be unevenly heated. The first few drops may feel fine, but the rest may be scalding hot.)

• Touch your baby's lip gently with the teat and wait for her to open her mouth. Don't try and force the bottle into her mouth: she knows when she is hungry.

• Hold the bottle as you would a pencil – and at almost the same angle. Try to keep the teat full of milk, to prevent her sucking in air. Resist jiggling the bottle to remind her it's there; her

sucking reflex will soon prompt her to start feeding – if she's hungry! Don't worry if she keeps stopping to rest; bottle-feeding is hard work for a small baby.

• If she starts spluttering and gasping take the teat from her mouth and sit her upright to get her breath. Tip the bottle up and check the flow of milk. It should be a slow drip. Using a slow-flow teat to start with will prevent her being overwhelmed by the flow of milk and encourage active sucking.

• If the teat starts looking squashed and your baby doesn't seem to be getting any milk, it may be that a vacuum has formed. Take the teat from her mouth for a moment, to allow air to enter the bottle. If this keeps happening, loosen the lid of the bottle slightly.

• When she stops sucking, gently ease the teat from her mouth. If there is milk left in the bottle, put a teat cover over the teat. If your baby has been feeding comfortably and has now

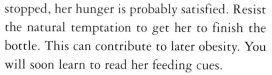
stopped, her hunger is probably satisfied. Resist the natural temptation to get her to finish the bottle. This can contribute to later obesity. You will soon learn to read her feeding cues.

• Give your baby a chance to bring up any swallowed air by sitting her gently upright or resting her against your shoulder. Rub her back very gently. If she has swallowed air, she will soon burp. It is normal for her to also bring up a small amount of milk. This is called 'posseting'. But, if she seems comfortable, don't disturb her. 'Winding' a baby is not always necessary.

• Sit and cuddle her for a while. She may be sound asleep and ready to lie down, or she may start filling her nappy. If she seems unsettled after having her nappy changed, she may want a little more milk. If only 10 minutes or so have passed, it's OK to give her some from the bottle you've just been using, but throw any leftovers away afterwards. This may seem wasteful, but once your baby has sucked on the teat, germs from her mouth will have contaminated the milk.

Other people feeding your baby

Every newborn baby needs to get to know one special person. Of course, there will be other adults who will hold her and sing to her sometimes – and these people may play a bigger part in her care as time goes by. But most experts feel that, to start with at least, a baby needs to identify with one individual who is there most of the time, protecting, loving and feeding. Secure in her attachment to this person, she will soon learn to love and trust others.

• Feed your baby yourself as much as you can. It is very easy to delegate bottle-feeding to others, but try not to do so for a while. Of course your partner or mother can give the occasional bottle while you have a break, but

STERILISING FEEDING EQUIPMENT		
Method	**How**	**Equipment needed**
Boiling	Boiling for 10 minutes Items remain sterile for several hours if the lid is not removed	Saucepan with lid
Steam	Steaming for 10 minutes Items remain sterile for several hours if the lid is not removed	You could use saucepan and steamer, but an electric steam unit is probably more convenient in the long term Expect to pay £25–£30
Chemical	Immersion in chemical solution for 30 minutes Items remain sterile so long as they are immersed (but solution must be renewed every 24 hours) Most health professionals recommend rinsing sterilised items with cooled, boiled water before use	Large tub or small bucket with a lid, or specially designed unit, plus sterilising tablets or liquid. Costs £12–£20 (A chemical reaction may occur if metal items are placed in the sterilising solution)
Microwave	Microwaving for 10 minutes Items remain sterile for up to 3 hours if the lid is not removed	Special unit to place inside microwave unit (Simply placing the items inside a microwave oven does not ensure complete sterilisation) Expect to pay about £10

resist pressure for most of her feeds to be given by other people. If you need to delegate, why not delegate something less fun – like cooking a meal or cleaning the bathroom?

How much milk?
Don't expect your baby to take much milk at all for the first few days. A newborn baby's stomach is about the size of a walnut – it doesn't take much to fill it.

As the days go by, her appetite (and her stomach) will grow. Feed her whenever she wakes and seems hungry, and let her decide how much milk she wants to take at each feed.

• Read the guidelines on the packet or tin of powdered baby milk. This will suggest how much milk to prepare for each feed.

• Let your baby decide when she has had enough – don't force her to finish the bottle simply to avoid waste.

• Don't expect her to take the same amount at each feed, or to feed at the same time each day.

• Don't expect her to sleep through the night for several months.

• If your baby seems restless soon after a good feed, try offering a little cooled, boiled water.

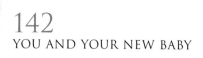

SPECIAL CIRCUMSTANCES

The journey from womb to world can be a tough transition for a baby and occasionally there are problems. On these pages we cover some of the situations that can arise.

During pregnancy, your baby was nourished and sustained by her placenta. The system worked smoothly for nine months until, suddenly, birth takes place and the umbilical lifeline is cut. From that point on, your baby is on her own; her heart no longer pumps blood to the placenta but redirects it to the lungs. A lack of oxygen forces your newborn baby to take a breath and, as the chest expands, air is sucked into her lungs.

The way her body does this is amazing: within just a short space of time, breathing, circulation and digestion are established and your baby is a separate little being. Sometimes, however, the process doesn't run so smoothly.

BREATHING DIFFICULTIES

Throughout pregnancy the placenta acts as your baby's lungs – delivering oxygen and removing carbon dioxide. Although she has been practising breathing movements since the eleventh week, her lungs contain fluid rather than air during pregnancy. This fluid helps keep the tiny air sacs open and unobstructed, ready for her first real breath.

As she passes down the birth canal, your baby's chest is squeezed and this fluid is eased out of her lungs into her mouth and throat. Her lungs are now poised ready for her first breath. When her body slips out of yours, the pressure on her chest is released, her lungs expand and air is drawn in. The respiratory control centre in

her brain clicks into action and she continues to breathe.

The fluid squeezed out of your baby's lungs will drain quickly away. Some midwives like to use a little suction gadget to remove this fluid, but this can be distressing for the baby, and is generally not necessary.

• Immediately she is born, keep your baby on her side or front, either across your tummy or in your arms. She may cough and splutter for a few seconds (and may swallow some of the fluid) but this will not hurt her. Cover her with your hands to keep her warm, and maybe rub her back gently. She will soon start breathing properly.

However, if your baby has passed meconium into the amniotic fluid during labour, your midwife may recommend immediate suction to remove any that may have entered her mouth. She may do this as soon as her head is delivered, to prevent your baby breathing in the meconium as she takes her first breath.

Sometimes, a baby's airways may be blocked by mucus, meconium or other fluids, and she may be unable to take that first breath until they are cleared. This may happen if she has been very short of oxygen during labour. Other factors may contribute to the problem. The birth may have been very traumatic, or the baby may be premature. There may be infection present, or a congenital problem.

If the baby was short of oxygen earlier in labour, the midwife will have recognised the signs and a paediatrician will be standing by to help. Occasionally the problem may not arise until the last few minutes before delivery. The baby will be born blue and weak, and the midwife will call for emergency help. She will start to suck fluid out from the baby's mouth and throat and, if experienced in doing so, she may use a use a special tube and light to enable deeper suction.

The doctor and midwife will work together to clear the baby's airways. To do this effectively, they will probably place the baby on a small resuscitation table to one side of the delivery room. She will be given oxygen through a small facemask. If she is still slow to breathe, air will be puffed gently into her lungs. This is called 'artificial respiration'. If necessary, the baby will be 'intubated' – a narrow tube will be placed down into her main airway to enable more efficient artificial respiration. Various drugs will be given to counter the effects of oxygen shortage.

Most otherwise healthy babies respond quickly and soon start to breathe without help. Provided the time without oxygen was not too long, there should be no further problems.

This situation is very distressing and frightening for everybody involved. You may not be able to see what is happening to your baby and the staff may, for a short time, be too busy to keep you informed. As soon as is physically possible, your midwife will return to your side and tell you what is happening.

It is usual for babies who have needed resuscitation to be taken to the Special Care Baby Unit (SCBU) for a few hours of close observation.

You should be able to hold and touch your baby before she is taken from the labour ward. Your partner could accompany her to the SCBU. Once your placenta is delivered, and all is well, ask to be taken to your baby.

FEEDING A SLEEPY BABY

Some babies may need to rest after a long or traumatic labour. Others may be sleepy and reluctant to feed because their mothers were given pain relief late in labour.

- Keep your baby close to you, ideally in bed beside you. Undress her to her nappy and hold her close to your bare breast. The smell and feel of your skin may soon prompt her to start feeding.
- Don't wait for your baby to cry before you try to feed her. By the time you have got organised, she may have got tired and fallen asleep again. Look for other signs that she is in a very light sleep and may be ready to feed: flickering of her eyelids, wriggling, small noises, mouth movements and 'rooting'.
- Hold her close to your breast and touch her lips with your nipple. Squeezing out a few drops of colostrum may also encourage her. But never force her head towards the breast. This kind of handling may cause long-lasting problems with breastfeeding.
- Consider having a bath with your baby. Lie back in warm water with your baby on your chest, her lower body in the water. Keep her warm by splashing her gently with water.

If your baby has not fed after 24 hours:
- Ask your midwife to show you how to express your colostrum. Doing this will help keep your supply going.
- If your baby is awake, but still drowsy and reluctant to breastfeed, you could give some of this colostrum to her. Discuss how to do this with your midwife: you could use a small cup, or a syringe. If you use a syringe, you may like to give your baby your index finger to suck at the same time (fingernail downwards – make sure it's cut short).

JAUNDICE

Throughout your pregnancy, your baby was dependent on the oxygen passed to her through the placenta and umbilical cord. Her blood contained extra red blood cells to transport this oxygen around her body. Once she has been born and has started breathing in oxygen through her own lungs, she no longer needs these extra red blood cells and her body starts to get rid of them.

This is what happens:

• The extra red blood cells are broken down in your baby's spleen (a large organ at the top of her abdomen). The main by-product of this process is a substance called unconjugated, fat-soluble bilirubin. Very high levels of unconjugated bilirubin are potentially toxic to cells, especially to the cells of the brain.

• The unconjugated bilirubin enters the blood stream, where it binds with protein molecules in the blood. As the level of unconjugated bilirubin in the blood rises, your baby's skin may become jaundiced.

• The unconjugated bilirubin is taken to your baby's liver where it leaves the blood stream. It is processed and converted into 'conjugated', water-soluble bilirubin. Conjugated bilirubin is not toxic.

• The conjugated bilirubin passes from your baby's liver, into her bile duct. This drains into her gut, and so the conjugated bilirubin passes out of her body in her faeces. As levels of unconjugated bilirubin in her blood fall, so your baby's jaundice will start to fade.

This is the normal process by which unwanted red blood cells are broken down and removed from the body.* It happens to all newborn babies, but only about 50% will become jaundiced. Because this jaundice is part of a normal body process it is often called 'physiological' jaundice. Physiological jaundice starts 2–5 days after birth and generally fades by the tenth day.

(*This process is happening continuously in all children and adults as old red blood cells are removed from the circulation to make way for new ones. However, except in newborn babies, it is happening at a very low level and does not generally lead to jaundice.)

If your baby becomes jaundiced

• Keep feeding your baby. Don't wait for your baby to cry: feed her when she seems ready (see 'Feeding a sleepy baby' page 143) – but don't wake her up just to feed. Research shows that forcing your baby to feed beyond her normal demands is of no benefit.

• Don't give any other fluids. If you give your breastfed baby other fluids, her tummy will be filled, and she will (quite naturally) not want to breastfeed. The passage of meconium through her body and removal of bilirubin may be even further delayed.

If levels of toxic unconjugated bilirubin become very high, phototherapy will probably be offered. The light from the phototherapy unit acts on unconjugated bilirubin in surface blood vessels, converting it to non-toxic conjugated bilirubin.

Your baby will be placed in her cot, naked except for her nappy and an eye patch to protect her eyes. A phototherapy unit will be positioned above the cot, so she is bathed in its blueish light. The light is pleasantly warm, and does not hurt. She may need phototherapy for a few hours or 1–2 days. She will remain next to your bed throughout this time.

Your baby will be very sleepy due to high bilirubin levels, but try to feed her at least every four hours.

If she is too sleepy to feed, ask your midwife to help you express some of your milk and give it to your baby using a cup or syringe.

Is my baby jaundiced?

• Examine your baby close to a large window so she is seen in daylight (colours often look different under artificial lights).

• The whites of her eyes are often the first part of the body to become yellow, followed by the skin of her face. If your baby has dark skin, it may be hard to see jaundice. Press the tip of her nose gently. The skin will blanch (become white for a second) and you will be able to see any yellowness.

• Take a look at the rest of her body. Your midwife may use a small colour gauge to assess the level of jaundice present. If very high levels are suspected, a sample of your baby's blood may be taken. Further tests will also be carried out to check for underlying problems such as infection or blood group incompatibilities.

Some babies become more jaundiced than do others. Jaundice that starts within the first 24 hours is not 'normal' jaundice, for example and will need special treatment.

HYPOGLYCAEMIA

Our bodies need glucose to function normally. If the level of glucose (a type of sugar) in our blood falls, our brains are the first body system to be affected. This is why we feel irritable and find it hard to concentrate when we get hungry. Extreme shortage of glucose may cause fits and brain damage.

Throughout pregnancy your baby is fed continuously through her umbilical cord and her blood glucose (sugar) levels remain fairly constant. Soon after delivery, the cord is cut and her body has to quickly adapt to cope with the resulting fall in blood glucose.

This is what happens:

• Less insulin is secreted (insulin is the hormone responsible for glucose metabolism).

• Glycogen, stored in her liver, is hurriedly brought in to be used in place of glucose.

• Ketone bodies, released from fat, serve as an alternative source of energy for the brain.

It is normal for a new baby's blood sugar levels to fall at times during the first 2–3 days of life. These three mechanisms will protect her from harm.

Try not to worry if your baby does not feed much in the first few days. Provided she is normal and healthy, she will not come to any harm. She does not need bottles of milk or sugar water. Nor does she need any blood tests to check her glucose levels.

Some babies, however, may be more vulnerable to this normal fall in blood sugar. This may be because their stores of alternative energy sources are low or have already been used up. Babies that need special attention include:

• Babies of diabetic mothers.

• Babies who have not grown well in the womb.

• Premature babies.

• Ill babies.

One of the signs of illness may be sleepiness and refusing to feed. This is why your midwife will keep a close eye on your baby until feeding is established. The things she will check for include:

• Raised temperature.

• Breathing difficulty.

• Early jaundice.

• Twitching or 'jumping'.

• Paleness.

Tell your midwife if you are anxious about your baby's appearance or behaviour.

If your baby is ill, she will be given the appropriate treatment – for example, antibiotics to treat an infection. There is still no need for her to be given a bottle. You will be helped to express off some colostrum and this will be given to your baby in a cup or syringe, or through a tube.

PREMATURE BABIES

A premature or 'pre-term' baby is one born before 37 weeks of pregnancy. Some babies are born as early as 28 weeks. Even a baby born this early has a 50:50 chance of survival. Babies as young as 24 weeks have survived and grown into healthy children.

Possible reasons for a pre-term birth include:
• 'antepartum haemorrhage' – part or all of the placenta becomes detached from the wall of the uterus, often because of pre-eclampsia (high blood pressure during pregnancy)
• serious illness in the mother – especially if she has had a high temperature
• multiple pregnancy and/or polyhydramnios (too much amniotic fluid)
• congenital problems, or rhesus incompatibility
• smoking, drug or alcohol abuse.

Often there is no obvious cause at all.

A pre-term baby has special needs. These will vary according to her age. A baby of 36 or even 35 weeks may not seem so very different from a term (40-week) baby, except that feeding may take a bit longer to get going. Younger babies, however, are very different and generally need special care.

In many ways, a very pre-term baby is not yet ready for life outside the womb – and so may need special technology to help her cope. She will probably be cared for in either a Special Care Baby Unit (SCBU) or a Neonatal Intensive Care Unit (NICU).

A pre-term baby may need help to:
• Keep warm. A very pre-term baby has very little fat and thin skin so she loses body heat very quickly. This is why she may be nursed in an incubator – to keep her warm. Special 'bubble-blankets' may also be used, and hats and socks will also help. Ask about 'kangaroo care' – warm skin-to-skin contact with you, too.

• Breathe. Her lungs may not be ready to work without help. She may need extra oxygen, maybe through a tiny tube taped to her nose. If she is very pre-term, she may need a tube in her airway and artificial respiration from a machine. A special monitor taped to her skin will measure the amount of oxygen in her blood, and an alarm will alert staff if she stops breathing for more than a few seconds. She may need drugs to help boost her blood circulation.
• Feed. A pre-term baby has smaller stores of energy than a full-term baby so she may have problems with low blood sugar unless she has regular feeds. If she is very pre-term, or she is having difficulty with breathing, she will not be able to suck – so she may be fed milk through a tube into her stomach. It won't be too long before she will be ready to try breastfeeding, or drinking from a cup or bottle. Pre-term babies need breast milk even more than term babies do. Even if you do not plan to breastfeed, please consider giving your pre-term baby your breast milk during her early weeks.

Your feelings

Most women who give birth prematurely feel very shocked and distressed. You may feel as though your world has been turned upside down. Your plans for pregnancy, birth and looking after your baby are suddenly overthrown and replaced with uncertainty and confusion. It is normal to feel disorientated and very, very anxious.

You may be shocked – even repulsed – by the appearance of your baby. She may seem bony and fragile and not at all cuddly. She may not even open her eyes to look at you. It is normal to feel a sense of deep loss and sadness for how things should have been.

If your baby needs special care, you may feel overwhelmed by the equipment and the number of people involved. You may feel incompetent

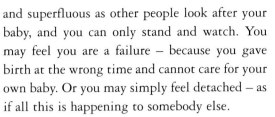

and superfluous as other people look after your baby, and you can only stand and watch. You may feel you are a failure – because you gave birth at the wrong time and cannot care for your own baby. Or you may simply feel detached – as if all this is happening to somebody else.

On the other hand, your baby's pre-term birth may be the welcome end of a difficult and uncertain pregnancy. You may simply be relieved and thankful that your baby is safely in your arms, even though she may still need special care for a while.

• Take things one day at a time. Accept your feelings as normal, and recognise that they will change as time goes by. It may help a lot to talk with somebody who has been through a similar situation. Ask the staff if there is a counsellor or support group for parents. The hospital chaplain may also be a great source of comfort and support. Contact your local NCT branch to find out if there is anybody on their Special Experience Register with whom you can talk.

• Keep in touch with your baby. Even a very tiny baby can be stroked and patted as she lies in her incubator. Talk softly to her: she will recognise your voice from her time in the womb. Ask if you can leave a small item of your clothing with her to remind her of your smell, and make sure you have a photograph of her to carry with you.

• Express your breast milk. The value of your breast milk cannot be underestimated – and this is something that you alone can do for your baby. Start expressing as soon as you feel well enough – ideally within the first 24 hours. Ask your midwife to show you what to do. She may give you a copy of UNICEF's leaflet *Expressing your Breastmilk* (otherwise available from UNICEF UK Baby Friendly Initiative, 20 Guilford Street, London WC1N 1DZ).

Don't forget: you are your baby's mother, whatever the circumstances and difficulties.

Although you may, for a time, need the help of others to care for her, you still have a unique and special bond with her that cannot be broken.

CONGENITAL PROBLEMS

One in every 20 babies is born with some sort of congenital problem. This may seem a lot, but remember that this figure includes everything from a minor birthmark, extra digit or small hernia – to major chromosomal disorders and abnormalities of the heart or brain.

However apparently minor the problem is, it is normal for you to feel very upset. It takes time to come to terms with the idea that your baby is different in some way from the one you imagined you'd have. At first, you may feel disbelief – it may all seem like a bad dream. You may feel guilt – and wonder if the problem was caused by anything you did or didn't do during pregnancy. You may feel angry – with your midwife, your partner, God – or your baby. All these feelings (and many others) are normal.

• Gather information. Ask to speak with the most senior person available.

• Get support. Telephone a helpline or contact a support group. Most women who do so say that just doing this helped tremendously. The Midwives' Information and Resource Service (MIDIRS) maintain a computer database of support groups. Contact MIDIRS on freephone 0800 581009 to find out details of an organisation that may be of help to you. Ring the NCT and ask for the Special Experience Register: names and phone numbers of women who are willing to support others going through a similar experience to their own.

• Give yourself time. Tell other people how you are feeling. Have a good cry, if this will help. Keep your baby close beside you. It may take time before you can see beyond her problem but, rest assured, that time will come.

A WATERBIRTH AT HOME

Sarah gave birth to her first baby, Ella, at home after seven hours labouring in a birthing pool. Marcus, Ella's father, joined them in the pool too, for the second stage of delivery.

When I told people I was planning a home birth they said I was either brave, irresponsible or mad. I didn't feel any of these; I just wanted to give birth in familiar surroundings and be able to collapse into my own bed afterwards with my husband and baby. But my GP advised me against the idea because of my age, nearly 35, the 15-mile drive to the hospital and the fact that it was my first baby.

I was very pleasantly surprised when my midwife accepted all my views on home births and actively supported me throughout my pregnancy. Even later on when I started reading about waterbirths and discovered I could hire a birthing pool to use at home she calmly told me she had delivered babies under water for nine years. However, she encouraged me to keep an open mind so that if something went wrong I would be prepared for admission to hospital.

'My midwife accepted all my views on home births and actively supported me throughout my pregnancy'

Eleven days before my due date I was as ready as I thought I could be: pool collected and assembled, TENS machine hired, home delivery pack ready and pethidine waiting in case I was desperate. We filled the pool half full to see how long it would take and wallowed in it for a while before emptying it – we didn't think we'd need it for at least a couple of weeks.

How wrong we were! The very next morning, after an evening of acute indigestion, I had a show and, as the day wore on, realised that labour had started. I spent the day vacuuming and preparing the bedroom and making sure my hospital bag was ready – just in case.

Afternoon

My husband, Marcus, moved the pool to a better position and spent four hours getting it filled and heated to the required 37°C – our kettle couldn't stand the pace and we had to borrow one from next door – well we were trying to heat 230 gallons of water!

When the midwife visited at 4.30pm she confirmed that I was in early labour and about 1 to 2cm dilated. She left saying that I had to get some sleep. Almost as soon as she left the contractions became stronger and more frequent and we only just managed to eat a light supper – sleep was out of the question. By 8pm I was keen to try the TENS machine but found it gave no relief whatsoever. Marcus gave me a back massage and we got the midwife back.

I was happy to learn that I was now 3cm dilated and to my surprise the midwife said I could get in to the pool. What amazing relief! The water was warm and soothing and my contractions were instantly more bearable.

Time passed and I lost all awareness of the world outside my living room. I wallowed in the water, listening to the conversations going on around me (we had been joined by a student midwife soon after I entered the pool), trying to eat yoghurt and dried fruit in between

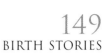

contractions and making sure someone changed the music on the CD player. Every 15 minutes the baby's heartbeat was checked – a condom on the end of the monitor kept it waterproof! The water temperature was monitored by using a floating beer thermometer.

Later that night

After two and a half hours I felt I needed more relief from the intensity of the contractions so the Entonox equipment was assembled. Once I'd got the hang of how to breathe in the gas and air, I found it helpful and I used it throughout the rest of the first stage. At about 2.30am I had to get out of the pool for an internal examination. This was when I realised the full effect of the water: on dry land it was much harder to find the right position to cope with the contractions and I was shocked to find what a difference it made. I was now 6 to 7cm dilated and making good progress.

'I can't describe the feeling of happiness'
says Sarah

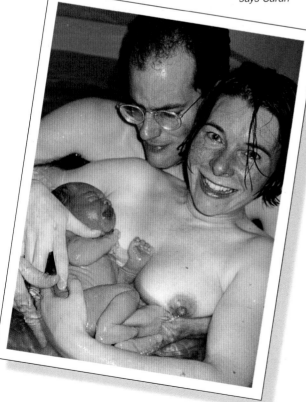

At 3am, after I had been in the pool just over four hours, I started feeling the urge to push – a whole new sensation which took me by surprise. A second qualified midwife was summoned and she arrived at 3.30am. Marcus then joined me in the pool and we decided the gas and air was no longer helping: it got in the way and I found it difficult to push and breathe at the same time.

Now that Marcus was in the pool with me I felt happier. He could hold me in the right position and help me stand up for the 15 minute heartbeat checks and I think he felt more useful.

The pushing stage lasted longer than it seemed at the time: nearly three hours. Towards the end I was starting to feel very frustrated as the

'In one splash she was born and lifted to the surface to breathe her first breath'

baby's head kept appearing and then disappearing completely. Then the head got stuck halfway and the midwives were about to ask me to stand up out of the water when I decided I had had enough: I gave one almighty push and out shot Ella – in one splash she was born and lifted to the surface to breathe her first breath. I had been in the pool for just under seven hours.

Delivery of the placenta took place out of the pool on a mattress on the floor. Ella helped by having her first feed. I didn't need any stitches.

Afterthoughts

If my birth plan had ever been written it would have read almost exactly as I have just described and I appreciate how lucky I am to be able to say that, because so many births don't go according to plan. I am sure the water helped, both for relieving pain and helping avoid the need for any stitches.

As for being at home, well I can't describe the feeling of happiness as I gazed at my new baby from the comfort of my own bed – accompanied by my husband and a cup of hot tea.

A SECOND HOME BIRTH

*Sarah and Steve's baby Abigail was born at home after a labour
that lasted through the early hours of a winter's morning just
before Christmas.*

During the last five weeks of the pregnancy I thought I'd gone into labour at least once a week, with really strong, regular contractions. My due date was 17 December, and I desperately wanted the baby to arrive before Christmas, but by 39 weeks I'd resigned myself to being pregnant well into the New Year.

2.30am

Several curries and long walks later, one morning two days before the due date, I woke up in a puddle at 2.30am, hissing at Steve to grab a towel (unprepared as usual, I didn't think it would happen to me, and hadn't covered the bed). My waters had broken, and I was quite excited that labour was finally starting, but there were no contractions so we tried to get some more sleep.

'I was quite excited that labour was finally starting'

About an hour later contractions started, but they were fairly few and far between. I decided to ignore them and dozed on and off.

Eventually I got up and wandered round the house to try and get things going. It worked, and an hour and a half later, when contractions were coming about every two to three minutes, I woke Steve and rang the midwife.

We had planned a second home birth without hesitation, as our first experience had been so relaxed and stress-free. We were both quite looking forward to doing another home birth all over again!

5.30am

The midwife arrived around 5.30am and we set up in the lounge. This included putting a plastic sheet over the sofa and floor, then covering it with an old bedspread. The midwife unpacked her equipment and made sure we had everything we needed. At this point, everything seemed to slow down completely, my contractions were further apart and not very strong at all, and I felt really silly for having called the midwife out too early. Anyway, I carried on pacing the floor, and finally the contractions started to come a bit stronger.

When our two-year-old, Anna, woke up at 6.30am Steve dressed her and she came downstairs and surveyed the scene. She didn't quite know what to make of it all, but enjoyed the fuss that was made of her, I think! I was still coping fairly well with the contractions at this point but during the next hour the contractions became even stronger and more intense. I needed to concentrate more and have Steve's help too, so a friend took Anna off to have breakfast, then sat with her in front of a video upstairs.

8.30am

Around 8.30am the contractions were getting on top of me a bit, I remember it suddenly dawning on me that I was going to have to push the baby out soon, and recalling the incredible pain of it the last time. However, by then there was no going back!

I started to use some gas and air which I found

helped enormously, even just having something else to concentrate on was really useful. Steve was sitting on the sofa, and I was kneeling on the floor, leaning on him while he supported me. After twenty minutes of very long, strong contractions, I began to push.

My second midwife, who had also delivered Anna, arrived only minutes before Abbie was born, with a student, who very helpfully held the camera and took lots of photographs.

The second stage lasted just three minutes, and as the midwife talked me through the process, I vividly remember feeling every part of Abigail's face being born, in great detail. I felt her head crown, followed by her nose, chin, and then the rest of her body

However, we were really pleased that Anna had been able to be involved, and that we hadn't had to disrupt her routine too much, or make her feel left out in any way.

I cut Abigail's umbilical cord (it was my turn, as Steve did it last time) and delivered the placenta naturally. I then went straight upstairs to the shower and let everyone else clear up the mess. Our friend whisked Anna off to her toddler group to break the news of Abbie's birth, and Steve made tea and toast.

'I cut Abigail's cord and delivered the placenta naturally'

Abigail's birth was a wonderful experience, I even enjoyed it! I felt so well that the next day we were all down on the quay in Exeter, feeding the ducks. Ten days later she slept through her first Christmas, with more presents than the rest of us put together.

Left: Big sister Anna meets her new baby
Below: Abigail was born screaming the place down

followed very quickly! She weighed 8lb 8oz, a whole pound and a half heavier than Anna, so I was quite surprised that her birth had been so easy. I was very grateful to have no stitches or tears.

Abbie was born screaming the place down, so when Anna came down to meet her new sister only minutes later, she wasn't very impressed, and soon went back to her video.

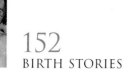
A BIG BOY BORN IN HOSPITAL

Lisa, an NCT breastfeeding counsellor, had hoped to give birth at home, but fears of pre-eclampsia meant that the decision was made to give birth to this baby in hospital.

Joshua was a planned home waterbirth, but the day before his due date, I went into hospital with high blood pressure and protein in my urine. The hospital was desperate to induce me, but I wanted to give things a chance to settle. My midwife agreed, but things did not improve, and eventually we decided that the baby really needed to be born. I was too worried about my older son to leave him staying with friends any longer. My midwife and I made the decision to try a homoeopathic induction, to see if that would get things moving. I was eager to avoid the doctor's idea of pessaries, a drip and an epidural because I wanted the birth to be as natural as possible.

'The hospital was desperate to induce me, but I wanted to give things a chance to settle'

The homoeopathic remedy got things moving: I had irregular contractions all night, and spent most of the night sitting up in a chair trying to get the baby to turn into an anterior position (i.e. with his back facing outwards). I was already three centimetres dilated before the remedy, so I hoped this would do the trick.

10am

By the morning, the baby had moved much further down and was in a good position but the contractions were weaker. We went into the delivery room, and Sharon, my midwife, broke the waters. She had convinced the doctors to give me a chance to get labour going without the syntocinon drip etc. I had my waters broken at about 10am.

Soon the contractions were regular and quite strong – about every five minutes. I was using my TENS machine and playing games to try and keep my mind off it. I had to stop to breathe with the contractions – still won the game though!

When the contractions became frequent, I started using gas and air. I found being on all fours to be the most comfortable position, leaning on Stuart (my partner) during the

Stuart cuts the cord

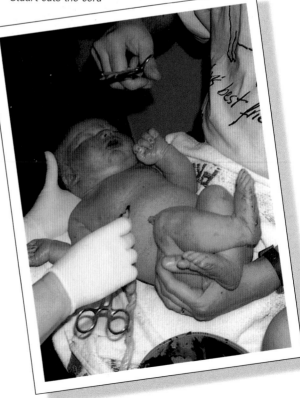

contraction, then moving back to all fours. I had expected to have a long labour, like my first, and was stunned to see Sharon getting everything ready. I managed to break the gas and air mouthpiece!

1pm

Soon Sharon asked me if I wanted to push (I'd made a pushy sound). I said 'no', then immediately 'yes'. I was sick at that point and the contractions actually stopped for about 10 minutes.

At that point, the gas and air (Entonox) just seemed to interfere with my concentration but I was hanging on to it like grim death just in case. I really had to push, I don't remember it being that intense with my first. It was incredibly painful not to push, and I was getting two or three pushes per contraction. I asked Stuart and Sharon if they could see anything yet as I could feel the head starting to crown. I put down my hand and felt the soft head. It was amazing and I cried with joy.

It was hard not to push when Sharon said to stop, and Stuart breathed with me. Then, with a push and a slither, the body was born. Stuart said, 'It's a boy', and Sharon passed him to me between my legs so that I could touch him.

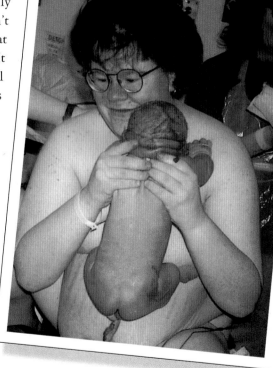

Joshua is lifted into the world to greet us

The labour had only been three and a half hours and the second stage only took about 20 minutes.

I could still feel the heaviness of the placenta, but had no urge to push. I wanted to have a natural third stage. We were all stunned at his size. He was so big. I picked him up and said, 'This is Joshua.' The cord was quite short and I had to be careful not to tug on it.

> **'I put down my hand and felt the soft head. It was amazing and I cried with joy'**

Joshua rooted and looked interested so I put him to the breast. I wanted to feed him as soon as I could and I knew that this would help with the third stage. I got an urge to push and quite quickly and easily pushed the huge placenta out.

Stuart cut the cord before it had finished pulsating. I am Rhesus negative and Sharon was eager to take the cord blood to test. When I was ready, Joshua was weighed and Stuart cleaned and dressed him. I needed three stitches. Joshua weighed an incredible 5.1kg (11lb 4oz).

We spent some time feeding and getting to know him. Someone brought my older son to the delivery room to meet his new brother. We had time as a family, then Stuart and Sharon took us back to the ward for the first hours of Joshua's life with us.

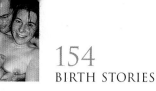
AN EMERGENCY CAESAREAN

Jack's birth did not go to plan. Although Sarah, his mother, is now grateful to have a happy, healthy toddler, she found the experience a shock that took some getting used to.

My pregnancy had been free of complications and, although I knew that one should be prepared for all eventualities, I didn't really believe that anything would go wrong when it came to the birth. With hindsight, there was some warning. From 36 weeks onwards, there was a question mark concerning the exact position of the baby's head. Was it engaged or not? No one was sure. I was told not to worry as it might not engage until the last minute anyway.

'My pregnancy had been free of complications and I didn't really believe that anything would go wrong when it came to the birth'

At 41 weeks, I went for a check-up at the hospital. I suspected that my waters had started leaking slightly that morning and this was confirmed. The doubt remained over the position of the head. I began to worry. I had read about low-lying placentas blocking the baby's exit, so I asked to see the consultant to find out once and for all what was going on.

The consultant felt my abdomen and announced calmly that the baby was in the breech position. I almost fainted from shock.

It was important that I had the baby within the next 24 hours, as leaking waters can give rise to infection. I had two options. I could have a caesarean now, or I could wait to see if I went into labour naturally within the next few hours. In the latter case, there would be 70% chance of a vaginal delivery. Failing spontaneous labour, I would need a caesarean. An induced labour was not an option as such labours can be too fast and furious for a baby in the breech position.

I was desperate to avoid a caesarean, so we went home and spent most of the day walking around the fields near our house, in an attempt to get things going. Nothing happened, and I was feeling very despondent. A caesarean was booked for the following morning. Then, that night, just as I was getting ready for bed, my waters broke dramatically.

Jack and Sarah straight after the birth

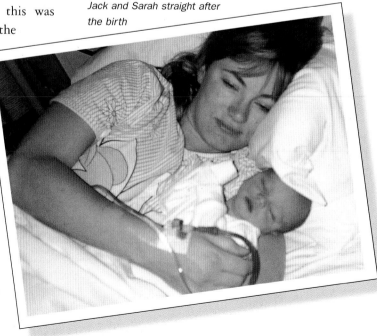

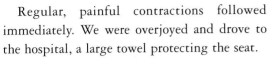

Regular, painful contractions followed immediately. We were overjoyed and drove to the hospital, a large towel protecting the seat.

As soon as we got there, the doctor carried out an internal examination. She said that I was five centimetres dilated. Then her face fell. She looked at the midwife, mumbled something about a prolapsed cord and pressed a red button above my head. A loud siren was activated.

The umbilical cord had passed through my cervix with the gush of the waters. It was now being squeezed dangerously with each contraction. I was told to get quickly on to my hands and knees. Then I was whisked down a corridor on the trolley, my backside in the air, while my bewildered husband ran alongside me. Throughout this, the midwife used her hand to keep the pressure off the cord, particularly during contractions.

I was taken into an operating theatre. My husband was no longer there. All around me, people were pulling on white boots, overalls and hats. Almost straight away, the anaesthetist put a needle into the back of my hand, and said that I would be asleep within a few seconds. Someone held a monitor against my stomach and announced, rather tactlessly, that she couldn't find the fetal heartbeat. I drifted into unconsciousness, resigned to the fact that I had lost the baby.

I was unconscious due to the general anaesthetic for about 45 minutes. During that time, my husband was taken to a side room and given tea and toast. A caesarean was performed without delay. The baby was examined and found to have Apgar scores of nine and then ten. In other words, he was in tip-top condition. If there is one person who did not suffer at all during Jack's birth, it was Jack himself.

When I regained consciousness, the first thing I saw was my husband sitting next to me, grinning and holding a little bundle. 'It's a boy!', he declared happily. Once I was convinced that the baby really was all right, I asked my husband to lay him next to me so that I could breastfeed him. He latched on like a natural and fed for half an hour.

'This had been both the worst and the best experience of my life. My emotions were in turmoil'

Everything seemed so strange. This had been both the worst and the best experience of my life. My emotions were in turmoil.

I remained in the hospital for just three days. Physically, I recovered very quickly. Emotionally, it took a lot longer.

I had been shocked by the speed of events and felt sad that my husband and I had not actually witnessed the birth of our son. However, I realise now that, while the birth is important, it is only the means to an end. The days, weeks, months and years following the birth are what really matter. Jack is now a lively, healthy and happy toddler. What more could I ask for?

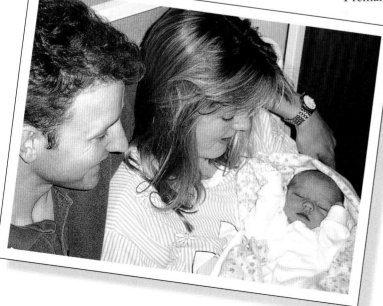

Happy new family

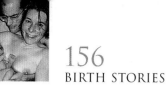
TWO CAESAREAN BIRTHS

Both Hannah's babies, first Riley and two years later, Miranda, were born by caesarean section. The first caesarean was unplanned and the second 'elective'.

At my first appointment with the midwife, when I was 16 weeks pregnant with Riley, the possibility of having a caesarean was suggested. The midwife asked me my height (5' 3"), shoe size (3 to 4) and height of my husband (6' 3"). Even at this stage, the midwife felt the proportions could lead to a caesarean but I put it down to old wives' tales – nothing I had read in the books had used such an arbitrary scale and no one in my family had had a caesarean.

> **'I just remember the relief and joy when our son Riley, was handed to me'**

At seven months, I saw the consultant at the hospital as part of my routine checks and he suggested I went for a pelvimetry (to measure the size of my pelvis) as he was concerned about the size of the baby and my proportions. No pressure was put on me by the medical staff and I resisted as I did not want x-rays scanning my unborn baby. However at 39 weeks, the baby's head had still not engaged, so I succumbed and made an appointment for the CT scan.

Riley

At 39 weeks, 4 days, I had a show in the early hours of the morning. I phoned the hospital at 8am and they said I should come to the hospital to be checked. When I arrived, I was put on a monitor and everything was quite calm and normal. Later on that day, I asked about the results of my CT scan and the consultant explained there was nothing unusual about the shape of my pelvis but the size was borderline and if I wanted to have a trial labour they would support me.

My husband visited me at the hospital after work at 6.30pm and within half an hour I started to go into labour naturally. I was moved into a delivery room and after eight hours of labour, gas and air, and a dose of pethidine, the consultant examined me and said I was 9cm dilated, the baby was in distress and still very high up.

3.30am

The anaesthetist was called and I was given an epidural – sudden relief from all the pain and contractions. It was now 3.30am the next morning and I was ready for the operating theatre to have an emergency caesarean section. My husband was kitted out in a green overall, hat and white wellingtons. As I had been in established labour for eight hours and under the effects of pethidine, I just remember the relief and joy when our son Riley, weighing 7lb 15.5oz, was handed to me. Everything seemed to happen so quickly and efficiently as shortly afterwards I was wheeled out of the operating theatre to recover, with patient attempts by the midwife to get Riley breastfeeding.

Before I left the hospital with Riley, the doctor, on her routine rounds, said that if I was thinking of having any more children (the last thing on my mind at the time!) I would need an elective caesarean birth. I did not feel cheated or felt I had missed out by giving birth this way.

I had at least given eight hours of labour a try and I did not experience an episiotomy, which I had convinced myself would be much worse.

Miranda

The arrival of Miranda, our second baby, by elective caesarean was a more planned event.

I arrived at the hospital at my appointment time, nine days before my due date. I saw the midwife who made sure my bowels were empty, shaved me then put me in a hospital gown. I went into the operating theatre accompanied by the anaesthetist as my husband was taken off to dress for the operating theatre.

I climbed on to the theatre table and I remember feeling cold and looking round to see the bright lights and the scalpels being wheeled to the other end of the table. The anaesthetist put a drip in my hand, switched on a few machines to monitor me and carefully placed the spinal block in my spine. To test the spinal block had taken effect, he asked me to lift one of my legs in the air every few seconds and fairly quickly, I lost all sensation and the surgeons got to work. Then, within ten minutes, the screen across the middle of my body was put down and I could see Miranda, weighing 6lb 15oz being delivered and she was handed to me straight away. It was wonderful to see her appear crying and I quickly forgot what was happening at the lower half of my body as the surgeons were stitching me up.

Miranda was taken away for a few minutes to be checked and weighed and then handed back to me warmly wrapped up.

Within an hour of entering the operating theatre, I was wheeled out and quickly established a position to breastfeed. Although I could only move the upper part of my body, I managed to find comfortable positions both sides to breastfeed Miranda. My husband and midwife were on hand to help.

After 24 hours, I was out of bed and trying to walk. Although painful at first, I recovered quickly and by the third day I could lift Miranda to feed and change her. I was in hospital for five

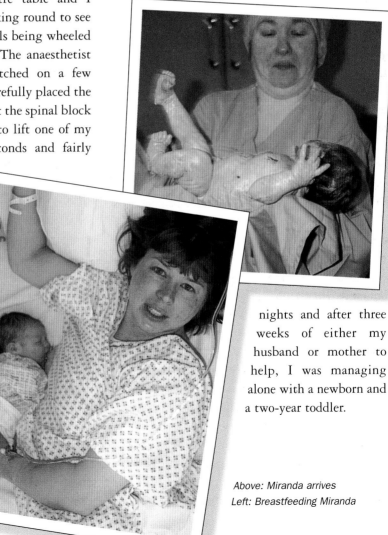

nights and after three weeks of either my husband or mother to help, I was managing alone with a newborn and a two-year toddler.

Above: Miranda arrives
Left: Breastfeeding Miranda

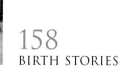

VAGINAL BIRTH AFTER CAESAREAN

After a first baby born at hospital and needing intervention, and a second baby born via a caesarean section, Hugh and Tikki's third baby, Sophie, was born at home in the usual way.

My first child, Ben, was born in hospital after a long and exhausting 36 hour 'on and off' labour, during which I couldn't sleep, and culminated in a forceps delivery. He had been in a posterior position. His birth was still a very positive experience.

Three years later, Rosie was booked to be born at home as I believed my body would work more efficiently where I felt safest. Unfortunately she was in the breech position and I felt safer going into hospital to have her. During labour she became distressed and needed an emergency caesarean section. Although I was disappointed, it was again a good experience and I made a quicker recovery than after Ben.

'I was sure that my body could do it'

Another three years on and Sophie was conceived. I knew she was to be our last baby and desperately wanted to give birth myself, without any technical help.

I did my homework: contacted the Caesarean Support Group, read all the relevant research and books, and really thought it through. Convincing the NHS that it was as safe as the research showed it to be, was rather difficult. Initially I was told that they would not provide me with care. They subsequently changed their minds but although they agreed to look after me, they were (as they admitted) inexperienced in 'vaginal births after a caesarean' (VBACs) and I was concerned that this might cause me to be unnecessarily admitted (albeit for the best of reasons). With this in mind, we cashed in a savings plan and 'opted out', employing an independent midwife who was experienced in home VBACs, Elaine.

I received first-class holistic care during my pregnancy and felt in safe hands. Elaine was very proactive about encouraging this baby into the optimum position, as she felt sure this would make a huge difference to the labour and birth.

Both my previous pregnancies had gone beyond 40 weeks, and this one was to follow the same pattern. At about 41 weeks Elaine explored options with me. I started using some acupressure on specific points, clary sage essential oil and all the others!

11.30pm

Two weeks over the due date, my contractions gently started during supper. We went to bed at the usual time but I found I wasn't really comfortable lying, so at 11.30 we got up, put on music and lit candles. Most of the time I stood and swayed/danced during contractions. I tried sitting astride a chair with Hugh massaging my back, but found I really wanted to be standing. I consumed a whole packet of Maltesers!

3am

By 3am my contractions were irregular but the odd one was very strong, so I contacted Elaine who said she'd get dressed and make her way over slowly. We were to page her if things speeded up. I relaxed into the birthing pool.

My contractions slowed right down and in the

30 minutes I was in the pool I only had four contractions. I didn't feel right in the water, much to my surprise; I felt I needed to be in contact with the ground.

I got out of the pool and considered going for a little walk down the road. However the contractions restarted with a vengeance and I couldn't stand, let alone walk! I settled myself on all fours leaning onto Hugh's lap while he massaged my back and generally held me.

3.45am

At about 3.45 I considered bleeping Elaine as I had just had a double-peaked contraction and knew deep down that things were progressing very quickly. At that point I remembered that our dog would have to be shut outside in his kennel and run, as he would bark when Elaine arrived and wake the children. Hugh went outside to construct a gate on the run in the pitch dark (we're not very organised). I had about three more very strong contractions and I discovered the analgesic properties of making a noise! Then my waters went. I called Hugh but he did not hear me. I went into auto-drive with just a hint of panic! I removed my pants and

tried to think which position might be best to deliver my own baby in. All of a sudden I felt Sophie move right down and immediately put my bottom in the air to slow what I felt was her imminent birth.

4.10am

At 4.10 I heard Elaine tapping at the door. Fortunately Hugh came back and let her in. Sophie's head was visible with each contraction. I found that I did not need to push. Elaine gave me the 'permission' to do whatever I needed to, and reassured me that what I was feeling was normal (as I had never felt a baby crown). She encouraged me to wriggle my hips, applied warm compresses to my perineum and intermittent pressure to my sacrum, all of which I found so useful.

5.10am

After a very gentle, calm, second stage Sophie was born at 5.10 to candle and firelight and the *Shoop Shoop* song (I hadn't had time to change the CD!) with me on all fours. The second midwife arrived just after the placenta had been delivered with the help of syntometrine as Elaine was a little concerned about my blood loss. I climbed back into the pool and relaxed there with a cool drink. Rosie and Ben both woke up and sat with Hugh, cuddling Sophie. My parents arrived (to look after the children while I was in labour) and joined us.

Later on, my sister and her son arrived and I have a wonderful photo of all of us squashed in together on our king-size bed. As far as Hugh was concerned, he loved the fact that we were in our own home and that he didn't have to leave us at all. It was the best £1,500 we've ever spent!

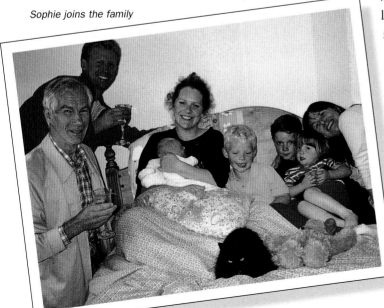

Sophie joins the family

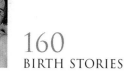

A BIRTH INDUCED IN HOSPITAL

Due to fears of pre-eclampsia, Safia and Alex's baby girl Denia was born after a fast labour which was induced in hospital – one week after her due date.

I was scheduled to give birth on 30 October and the final few weeks leading up to that date had passed very slowly. My fiancé, Alex and myself were feeling both nervous and excited at the same time. The due date came and went with no sign of the baby who was obviously far too cosy in my tummy. On Thursday 4 November during my check-up, too much protein was found in my urine and I was asked to go home, collect my maternity bag and return to the hospital for observation and induction over the following few days.

'The due date came and went with no sign of the baby'

My mum had arranged to come from France for only a few days so I was hoping to be induced while she was in the country. I picked her up at Waterloo Station, collected my bag and then checked myself into the hospital. I was feeling frustrated about being in hospital but realised it was for the best as myself and baby were being monitored for the possible signs of pre-eclampsia. I had been suffering from mild headaches and sometimes had flashing lights in my head.

Friday came and went with my mum by my bedside all day, then Alex joined me in the evening after work. There were still no signs of our baby wanting to put in an appearance. Saturday was similar though my parents-in-law and my boss visited me, which definitely helped to relieve the boredom.

I never thought that I would be hospitalised just prior to giving birth, so I was a bit apprehensive. Being in an unfamiliar environment combined with the pressure of not knowing if everything was going to be fine or not, was rather difficult. I really wanted to be at home, so much that I kept asking the midwives if I could be discharged and go home to rest. The midwives quite rightly told me that they didn't want to hear me say the 'H' word again. On no account were they about to let me go home! On Saturday evening however, the doctor planned an induction for the following day. The long nine-month wait was almost over.

On Sunday morning I was about to take a shower when the midwife told me to pack my things and move to the labour ward. I called Alex and my mum to tell them the induction was going to start later that morning.

10.45am

At 10.45am, pessaries were introduced and I was told that labour could either commence very quickly or that it could be a long wait for me, with my baby deciding to come as late as the following Tuesday. I was due to be checked over six hours later and was sent back to wait in the ward.

In the early afternoon I managed a small amount of food and a quick sleep. Since the pessaries had been introduced I was starting to feel my muscles move and start to dilate. Something was beginning to happen!

2pm

I had a bath and Alex rubbed my back as I was starting to feel pain and by 3pm I was having agonising contractions which were frequent and intense.

Françoise, my mother-in-law, could clearly see that labour had started very fast so she asked the midwife to check on me and give me some painkillers. When the midwife checked, I had dilated two to three centimetres so I was sent straight to the labour ward where she explained that the process could still last a long time.

During my pregnancy, I had decided to have a natural childbirth, but with the onset of severe pain, all of those plans changed. I would have taken any form of painkiller they had offered me! By now the pain was excruciating and it was making me feel weak. I really thought at that moment that I wouldn't be able to cope with the imminent birth.

I asked for an epidural for which they prepared me. However, the baby's heart rate was fluctuating too much and the hospital had unfortunately forgotten to send a sample of my blood to the laboratory for testing. While I was waiting for the team to decide if it was wise to administer an epidural, I relied on gas and air, which I initially refused, but then totally relied upon as the contractions continued.

Alex was next to me every step of the way and his presence was essential as it really reassured me that everything was going to be fine.

5.30pm

It became obvious to the delivery team that I was too far advanced to have an epidural and the pain seemed now almost unbearable. The baby's heart rate was fluctuating too much by now which led the

'I had decided to have a natural childbirth, but with the onset of severe pain, all of those plans changed'

delivery team to prepare me for a caesarean section. The doctor explained that she may have to take a sample of blood from the baby's head. However, it was at this moment I felt the urge to push and entered the second stage of labour. The doctor checked on me and found to her surprise that I had dilated to nine centimetres, much faster than anticipated. In fact I had dilated from three to nine in the space of half an hour!

After several intense minutes of pushing and with the help of cries of 'push!' and 'you're nearly there!' from Alex, baby Denia's head appeared. Another push later and I felt her body come out. I knew she had arrived when I heard a cry. The time was 6.01pm and it had only been three hours and one minute of contractions. Within minutes she was in my arms.

All was not quite over however as the placenta was then delivered and I had to have a few internal stitches, but it didn't really matter as I was feeling overwhelmingly happy and emotional.

Alex and Safia meet Denia at last

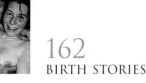

GIVING BIRTH TO TWINS

A twin birth can be a tricky one, but Debbie, herself an experienced midwife, knew what her options were and gave birth to her two babies in a hospital birthing pool just before their due date.

I approached the birth of my twins with a mixture of excitement and trepidation. I had confidence in my ability to give birth following a waterbirth at home with my first child but discovering at 20 weeks that my second pregnancy was to be twins added more than a degree of uncertainty.

Unable to find any research on the safety of twin home births I resigned myself to a hospital delivery. I was lucky enough to have a wonderful community midwife Carole who provided all my ante-, intra- and postnatal care. I trusted her implicitly and without her support could never have achieved such a positive experience.

I enjoyed a very healthy pregnancy, working until 28 weeks, practising yoga and swimming throughout. The babies grew well and were both presenting head first. I saw my consultant twice, the latter appointment at 34 weeks to discuss my birth plan. I emphasised that in the absence of complications I wished to have privacy in which to labour, minimal intervention and monitoring, a natural and active birth, using water for labour and delivery of the first baby and a physiological third stage. He was extremely supportive and having discussed and written down these preferences, I was able to relax and look forward to the birth.

'I was lucky enough to have a wonderful community midwife. I trusted her implicitly and without her support could never have achieved such a positive experience'

9pm

Labour started two days before my due date with a bout of excessive fetal movement and generalised discomfort around 9pm. Contractions were quickly established between three and eight minutes apart but I waited an hour before calling my midwife as, although I was excited, I could hardly believe it had really started. By 11.30pm, labour was well established and Carole came to our home to find me kneeling against my husband Ian and concentrating hard on my breathing. We all transferred to hospital without further ado, the car journey being better than I'd imagined. The room prepared for me was warm and dark and quiet. The move from home had been unsettling but once there I switched off from the outside world and concentrated on giving birth.

'The move from home had been unsettling but once there I switched off from the outside world and concentrated on giving birth'

The pool was run and I had the short fetal heart monitor I'd agreed to, held on by Carole rather than tightly strapped on, for which I was grateful. I'd hoped my cervix might be four to five centimetres dilated and was staggered when an internal examination revealed I was already nine centimetres.

The water was lovely. It didn't take the pain away but helped me to cope with it. The buoyancy was a welcome relief and enabled me to change positions easily, settling into a half kneeling, half squatting position for both births. I also appreciated the sense of privacy the pool gave me, especially as twin deliveries often attract a large audience. Carole, a supporting midwife, and my husband were my only attendants, the consultant and paediatrician tactfully hovering nearby in the corridor.

1am

My waters broke spontaneously as I went into second stage and I felt the first baby moving down. I didn't have a strong urge to push but doing so relieved the pain a little and at 1.17am, after 20 minutes of noisy pushing, my baby son was born into the water. I delivered him myself bringing him gently up to the surface.

It was an extraordinary moment, holding my baby safely in my arms but, knowing that I had to do it again, I felt euphoria overridden by continuing pain and uncertainty regarding the second and often more complicated birth.

Holding the baby with the cord still attached I left the pool as we agreed and lay on a mattress to be re-examined and have the presentation confirmed. I was restless and in pain so when it was announced that all was well, I didn't need asking twice if I'd like to go back into the pool. The second bag of waters broke spontaneously and I felt the baby coming. In spite of my vocal protests there was nothing I could do to prevent my daughter being born in two reluctant but much easier pushes, 17 minutes after her brother. Again I brought her to the surface but she didn't cry as readily and spent a moment being vigorously dried and 'pinked up' with some oxygen before yelling her objections.

> 'It was an extraordinary moment, holding my baby safely in my arms but knowing that I had to do it again'

As I had a minimal blood loss, I went ahead with a physiological third stage and pushed the placenta out kneeling on the floor nine minutes later.

The babies were healthy: Joe weighing 7lb 5oz and Faye 6lb 11oz. They both breastfed and we went home the same morning. I had achieved a safe and natural twin waterbirth which filled me full of a sense of achievement and pride, with gratitude to my carers, and love for my babies – a truly positive birth experience.

Debbie with twins Joe (right) and Faye (left)

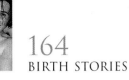

A LITTLE SISTER BORN AT HOME

Belinda and Nigel had a third little girl, born at home one beautiful summer's day, after a busy morning at the swimming pool and the burger bar.

'Well, you are two centimetres dilated!' Lynn, my midwife, pronounced at my antenatal visit, three days after my due date had passed. I was surprised because I had not felt anything that might remotely be called a contraction.

'The baby might come today!' I told my two older daughters – who went wild with excitement. But two more days came and went still with no contractions that I could detect.

'Four centimetres dilated and I can feel the membranes and the baby's head,' said Lynn, five days after my due date.

'It's a good job I'm having this baby at home,' I said 'because if I wasn't I'd have been told I was failing to progress and would have been induced!' Lynn laughed – but we both knew it was true.

'Well it won't be long now – hope you have everything ready,' she added.

I muttered that the baby would have to wait till after we had been swimming and been for a burger as promised to my 4- and 7-year-olds.

'I muttered that the baby would have to wait till after we had been swimming and been for a burger as promised to my 4- and 7-year-olds'

12.15pm

It wasn't until we were leaving the swimming pool at 12.15 that I was sure that I felt a contraction. But the moment it passed I was convinced I had imagined it. At MacDonald's I surprised the lad who was serving me by leaning on the counter and gasping out my burger request. It was 1pm. Luckily the children were persuaded to have a take-away. I wanted a home birth not a burger-bar one! Home, after a longer than usual pause at a roundabout to let a contraction pass, I called Nigel, my partner, just as another contraction arrived. This shocked him into a very fast trip home!

2.15pm

When Nigel walked in 20 minutes later I was calmly drying my hair and the children were watching a video. As an old hand at home births (daughters one and two were both born at home) he swung into action changing the bed and running a bath. We chatted about arrangements. At 2.15 I stepped into a deep, warm bath and called the midwife on the mobile. 'Well I'll just finish these couple of visits then I'll be over – just time the contractions for me.'

I put the phone down and timed – five minutes to the next one then a gap of four then three then two minutes and increasing length and pain with each one. I called back – 'I think you need to come now!' I said. Children were told and came to kiss me goodbye as they left for the childminder. Lynn arrived at 2.45pm and told me I was eight centimetres dilated.

Out of the bath and into the bedroom. 'Would you like some Entonox?' Lynn fumbled with the cylinder and gas escaped – she and Nigel fought the cylinder. It would have been funny if I had not been so keen to have a whiff of gas!

Entonox doesn't seem to relieve the pain, it just makes you too high to care. I noticed the window was open on this lovely summer day and wondered what the neighbours thought of my yells and repertoire of swear words.

The pain seemed to be about the same as with the other two births but just compressed into a shorter time space!

The second midwife arrived and introduced herself. She was a hospital midwife and this was her first home birth where she was the supporting midwife.

My world had shrunk to me, the midwives and Nigel. There was barely a gap between contractions. All the time Lynn was encouraging me and filling me with confidence – her colleague likewise – in looks, touches and words.

'Relax your bottom,' she said. Relax your bottom when you feel you are about to poo a giant prickly football! How? I thought. But she rubbed me and reminded me that I was doing

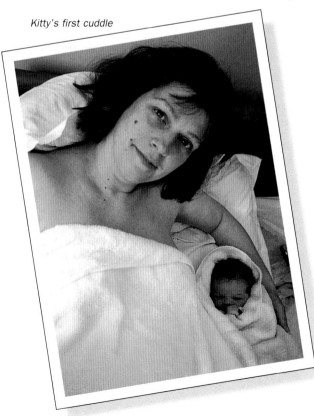

Kitty's first cuddle

brilliantly and I relaxed, the pain eased and suddenly I wanted to move from all fours to a semi-sitting position.

We seemed suspended in a moment free from pain. Then another contraction and this time, with no voluntary decision from me, a tremendous but painless push.

3.30pm

Then a space. I pulled myself up and said to Lynn, 'I don't want to do this any more.'

'Well you can't go to Sainsbury's like this – look, your baby's head is here.' I was stunned. Lynn smiled and a second involuntary push and the baby was out and lifted warm and wet on my tummy, not crying just blinking in the light. It was 3.40pm.

> 'I noticed the window was open and wondered what the neighbours thought of my yells and repertoire of swear words'

Within 15 minutes the children were back to see their baby sister and to help me dress her for the first time. Nigel called relatives and answered one business call: 'No, she can't speak to you right now, she's busy – she's just had a baby – yes a baby – here, about 15 minutes ago!'

The midwives melted away taking their equipment with them and we were left in peace to get used to being a family of five. It was a perfect summer's day.

Later, when all five of us were tucked up in the double bed, my four-year-old was talking to her Grandma on the phone: 'We had a busy day: we had a burger and we went swimming and we went to the doctor's and we watched a film at the childminder's and had pizza for tea – oh and mummy had a baby too.'

Postscript – the second midwife attending the birth decided to move to work in the community so she could have the opportunity to take part in more home births.

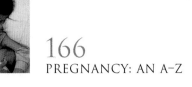

PREGNANCY: AN A–Z

If your midwife, GP or antenatal class teacher isn't available to answer your queries, we hope this A–Z list of common terms will help. Do consult a health professional if anything worries you.

ACTIVE BIRTH

Being active may make labour shorter and more comfortable. Many women find that remaining upright and mobile, walking around during the early stages, and using different positions to ease the pain makes labour easier to cope with.

AFP TEST

Screening blood test carried out between 16 and 18 weeks of pregnancy. Measures the amount of Alpha-Feto-Protein in your blood. High levels mean the baby is at risk of spina bifida and low levels, of Down's syndrome. If your AFP is high or low, further tests such as a detailed ultrasound or amniocentesis will be suggested.

AFTERBIRTH

➤ PLACENTA

AFTERPAINS

Contractions that occur after the baby has been born and help the womb regain its pre-pregnancy size. Some women may find them painful. They are more commonly felt after second babies than first. Homoeopathic arnica tablets may help with the discomfort, or you may wish to take paracetamol for a day or two. They are often at their strongest during breastfeeds.

AIDS

Acquired Immunodeficiency Syndrome which may develop some years after infection with the HIV virus. AIDS means that the immune system is so weak that the patient cannot fight off infections such as pneumonia which cause serious illness or death.
➤ HIV

ALLERGIES

Sensitivity to various foods, dust, animal fur or other environmental factors. Babies receive some protection against allergies leading to asthma and eczema if they are breastfed exclusively (i.e. without being given any formula milk) for four months and not given solid food until 15 weeks (Dundee Infant Feeding Study 1998, *BMJ*, A. Wilson *et al.*).

AMNIOCENTESIS

Test to diagnose spina bifida, Down's syndrome and other genetic disorders. Carried out between 13 and 20 weeks of pregnancy by putting a needle through the mother's abdomen and drawing off some of the amniotic fluid. Baby cells in the fluid can be examined, to confirm the presence of specific genetic disorders like Down's.
➤ AMNIOTIC FLUID

AMNIOFILTRATION

Specialised pregnancy test carried out at 12 weeks. A needle is used to remove amniotic fluid from the womb. The baby's cells are filtered out of this fluid and cultured in the laboratory to test for abnormality. Immediately after filtration, the fluid is replaced in the womb.

AMNIOTIC FLUID

The fluid in which the baby floats during pregnancy. Also called 'waters' and 'liquor'. Amounts to 0.5 to 1.5 litres by the eighth month. Too little (oligohydramnios) may indicate problems with the baby's urinary tract; too much (polyhydramnios), problems with the oesophagus or spinal cord.

AMNIOTIC SAC

The 'bag' which lines the womb and contains the baby and the waters. It consists of two membranes, the chorion or outer layer, and the amnion which is closest to the baby.

ANALGESIA

Medical name for pain relief. Gas and air (Entonox), TENS, pethidine (Meptid, diamorphine) and epidurals are examples of labour analgesia. Having a bath, changing position, and controlling your breathing are also forms of pain relief.
➤ ENTONOX; EPIDURAL; PETHIDINE

ANTERIOR POSITION

An anterior or occiput-anterior (OA) position is when the baby lies with the back of his head facing the front of your pelvis. Labour tends to be shorter and less painful when the baby is occipito-anterior.

ANTIBIOTICS

Must be used with caution during pregnancy, as many have adverse effects on the baby. Never dose yourself with antibiotics left over in your medicine cupboard. Doctors sometimes prescribe safe antibiotics to pregnant women with bladder or vaginal infections as these can cause premature labour.

ANTIBODIES

Proteins made by your body to fight off infections – for example, rubella antibodies protect against rubella (German measles). Blood is taken for antibody screening at your first antenatal check, and again at 28 weeks and possibly 32 weeks. You pass some antibodies, and therefore some protection from these infections, on to your baby. Maternal antibodies wear off during the first few months of the baby's life.
➤ GERMAN MEASLES

ANXIETY

Causes your body to produce stress hormones such as adrenalin. Too much adrenalin may be bad for your baby, so relax and enjoy your pregnancy. It also slows labour down, and this is why antenatal classes teach relaxation techniques.

APGAR

A score out of 10 to measure how strong your baby is one and five minutes after birth. Points are given for heart rate, breathing, muscle tone, reaction to stimulus and skin colour. The midwife who helps you deliver your baby will make a quick visual assessment and then note it down. At birth, a baby might typically score 7 and five minutes later, 10. A low Apgar score may mean your baby needs some extra care. A paediatrician may be called to check him over.

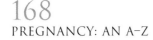
AREOLA

The coloured circle of skin around your nipple. During pregnancy, you might notice raised areas on the areola. These are called Montgomery's tubercles and secrete substances to keep the nipple supple. When breastfeeding, most of the areola should be in your baby's mouth.

AROMATHERAPY

Aromatherapists treat people with essential oils made from plants. When inhaled, also taken in through the skin in massage etc., the oils cause the release of healing chemicals into the blood stream. Many essential oils are dangerous during pregnancy and labour, so consult a qualified aromatherapist before trying them.

BACKACHE

Common during pregnancy, because the weight of the baby drags the spine out of shape and pregnancy hormones soften the ligaments that hold the back of the pelvis in place. Stand tall, keeping your back as straight as possible. Backache in labour can be relieved by using an all-fours position.

BART'S TEST

Screening test developed at St Bartholomew's Hospital in London, and now widely available. Blood is taken at 16–18 weeks of pregnancy and two, three or four substances are measured to assess the baby's risk of Down's syndrome or spina bifida.

BLOOD PRESSURE

An important indicator of your health during pregnancy. The midwife records two figures in your notes (e.g. 120/70) by wrapping an inflatable cuff around your arm. A raised lower figure is one possible indicator of pre-eclampsia.
➤ PRE-ECLAMPSIA

BONDING

The special relationship between a mother and her new baby that develops in the first hours and days of the baby's life. Being close to the baby, and especially having skin to skin contact, seems to promote maternal behaviour.

BRAXTON HICKS CONTRACTIONS

Towards the end of pregnancy, you may notice occasional contractions when your tummy tightens and feels very hard. These contractions are not painful. Some women have quite a lot and others none at all.

BREATHING EXERCISES

If you go to antenatal classes, you will learn how to use the rhythm of your breathing to help you cope with pain in labour. Breathing exercises form the basis of yoga and many other relaxation techniques.

BREATHLESSNESS

Often a problem in late pregnancy when you have a lot of extra weight to carry around and lung space is restricted. Women whose babies are in the breech position may be especially breathless because the baby's head presses against the diaphragm.

BROW PRESENTATION

An abnormal presentation in which the baby's neck is stretched so the front of the head is the presenting part rather than the back. Since the brow is wider than the back of the head the baby cannot fit through the pelvis and a caesarean is necessary.

CARPAL TUNNEL SYNDROME

Swelling in the narrow passageway which carries nerves from your wrist to your hand can cause pressure on the nerves which could result in pins and needles and numbness of your fingers. This sometimes happens in pregnancy due to fluid retention. Resting with your hands raised, exercises or wrist splints can all help. It will usually settle after the birth.

CEPHALIC

Sometimes abbreviated to ceph. This is the usual position for a baby in the uterus, with the head pointing downwards.

CEPHALO-PELVIC DISPROPORTION (CPD)

This occurs if the baby's head is too big to get through your pelvis. CPD is sometimes diagnosed antenatally using ultrasound or x-rays, but more often during labour when the baby does not move down through the pelvis. A caesarean section is necessary.

CEREBRAL PALSY

The causes of cerebral palsy are currently under investigation; the result is a baby who may be born with physical and mental disabilities. People with cerebral palsy used to be called spastics.

CERVICAL INCOMPETENCE

A condition leading to miscarriage when the muscles of the neck of the womb (cervix) are so weak that the cervix starts to open early in pregnancy. Women with this problem may have a stitch put in the cervix to keep it closed. This stitch is called a Shirodkar suture.
➤ CERVIX; SHIRODKAR SUTURE

CERVICAL MUCUS

Lubricates the vagina. It becomes thinner and more plentiful when you ovulate. Examining the mucus can help you decide when is the best time to try for a baby.

CERVIX

The neck of the womb. It is long, hard and tightly closed during pregnancy. At the start of labour, it becomes softer and shorter and then gradually opens until it is 10cm dilated.

CHLAMYDIA

An infection caught through sexual intercourse. Although the woman may have no symptoms, the presence of the infection in the vagina can lead to premature labour. It can also cause problems with the baby's health.

CHLOASMA

An increase in the pigmentation of the skin on the face which can cause a mark to appear on the cheeks. It is sometimes called a 'butterfly mask'. It disappears after the baby is born.

CHORIONIC VILLUS SAMPLING (CVS)

Diagnostic test carried out at around 11 weeks of pregnancy to find out whether the baby has Down's syndrome. Under ultrasound guidance, a needle is passed through the mother's abdomen and a sample of the placenta taken.

COLOSTRUM

The thick yellowish milk produced in small quantities by your breasts before the mature milk comes in. It is rich in antibodies and protects your baby against many diseases.
➤ ANTIBODIES

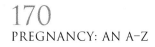

CONSTIPATION

Often caused by pregnancy hormones slowing the passage of food through the large bowel, and also by iron tablets. To avoid it: eat plenty of roughage, fresh fruit and vegetables. If taking iron, ask your doctor for a different prescription.

CONTRACTIONS

Tightenings of the muscles of the womb that occur throughout a woman's fertile years, but which become much stronger during labour when they open the neck of the womb and push the baby out into the world.

CORDOCENTESIS

Specialised pregnancy test, carried out under ultrasound guidance, which involves taking blood from the baby's umbilical cord. The blood is examined to see if the baby has haemophilia, anaemia, problems with his immune system or other abnormalities.

CRAMP

Leg cramps are common during pregnancy. Drinking plenty of milk may help reduce the frequency of attacks. If you have a cramp, flex your foot firmly upwards, then circle your ankle vigorously.

CYSTITIS

An infection of the bladder which leads to frequency of passing urine and pain. Cystitis should always be treated with antibiotics to prevent the infection from spreading to the kidneys. Drink plenty of water to help wash the infection out. Some research suggests that drinking cranberry juice may also help relieve the symptoms.

DEEP TRANSVERSE ARREST

This complication of labour occurs when the baby cannot get past the two bony projections that protrude into the pelvis. Sometimes, a caesarean is necessary, or forceps may be used to turn the baby's head so that it can pass the spines.

DIABETES

Failure of the pancreas to produce insulin causes sugar to accumulate in the blood leading to extreme thirst, drowsiness and eventually coma. Some women develop pregnancy diabetes but doctors are unsure whether this should be treated like ordinary diabetes. Babies of diabetic mothers can be very large. Your urine will be tested for sugar at antenatal check ups.

DOMINO SCHEME

Pregnancy care is provided by your GP and a community midwife or small group of midwives. When labour starts, one of the midwives accompanies you to hospital and helps you give birth, returning home with you and the baby 6–8 hours later. It is only available in a few areas.

DOULA

A Greek word meaning 'wise woman'. Used to describe an experienced mother who supports another woman during labour, and helps her care for her baby during the first few days at home.

DOWN'S SYNDROME

Sometimes called Trisomy 21, this syndrome is caused by an abnormal twenty-first chromosome. People with Down's are of below average intelligence and may have heart and lung problems. Many, however, can achieve independence with some support in their adult lives, though the degree of disability varies greatly.

DUE DATE

Correctly referred to as 'estimated date of delivery' (EDD). Your due date is nine months and one week from the first day of your last menstrual period. Remember that most babies are not born on their due date!

ECLAMPSIA

A serious medical condition, usually preceded by pre-eclampsia, when the mother has major fits similar to those of epilepsy. These can occur during pregnancy, labour or in the postnatal period. The mother requires treatment in an intensive care unit.
➤ PRE-ECLAMPSIA

ECTOPIC PREGNANCY

An ectopic pregnancy is one that occurs outside the womb. The fertilised egg embeds in the Fallopian tube or occasionally, in the abdomen. If it embeds in the tube, the mother experiences severe pain, followed by miscarriage, haemorrhage and often the loss of her tube.

EDD – ESTIMATED DATE OF DELIVERY

➤ DUE DATE

EFFLEURAGE

A form of massage which involves stroking the skin with the fingertips to stimulate the nerve endings that respond to light touch. Effleurage of the tummy can be comforting in labour.

EMBRYO

The name given to the unborn baby from conception to the end of the third month of pregnancy – after that it's a fetus.

ENDOMETRIUM

The inner lining of the womb (uterus). There are two other layers – the myometrium or muscle layer and the perimetrium or outer covering. It is the endometrium that is shed each month when you have a period.
➤ UTERUS

ENEMA

Used to be given routinely to women in early labour to empty the back passage and so make more room for the baby in the pelvis. Rarely used nowadays since it is recognised that most women tend to have diarrhoea at the beginning of labour and don't need one.

ENGAGEMENT

When the baby's head or bottom sinks down into the pelvis during the last month of pregnancy. If your baby is four-fifths engaged, the midwife can feel only one fifth of his head above the bony cage of the pelvis.

ENGORGEMENT

Your breasts feel hot, hard and uncomfortable due to a surplus of milk. If your baby finds it difficult to latch on, express a little milk by hand to make your breasts softer. Usually, engorgement isn't a problem after the first few weeks of breastfeeding.

ENTONOX

A mixture of 50% oxygen and 50% nitrous oxide which can be inhaled by the mother during labour for pain relief and is always under her control. In hospitals, it is usually piped into

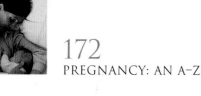

delivery rooms from a central source. Can be supplied in cylinders for a home birth.

EPIDURAL

The nerves supplying the uterus and cervix are anaesthetised by injecting a pain killing solution around the spinal canal below the spinal cord, removing all sensation from the waist downwards. Low dose or 'mobile' epidurals are now being developed to provide pain relief with some mobility.

EPISIOTOMY

A cut made through the back wall of the vagina into the perineum to enlarge the opening so that the baby can be born more easily, or so that forceps can be placed around the baby's head.
➤ PERINEUM

EXTERNAL CEPHALIC VERSION (ECV)

If your baby is breech at the end of pregnancy, your consultant may try to turn her by placing one hand on her head and one on her bottom and pushing her round. A succesful external version may avoid the need for a caesarean section.

FALLOPIAN TUBE

The tubes (one on each side) that connect your ovaries to your womb and where fertilisation of the egg by the sperm takes place. Tiny waving hairs in the walls of the tube propel the egg onwards towards the womb.
➤ FERTILISATION

FALSE LABOUR

Many women find that Braxton Hicks contractions become more frequent towards the end of pregnancy, and can sometimes be painful. They may interpret this as the start of labour, but unless the contractions are causing the cervix to soften and open, it is a 'false' alarm.
➤ BRAXTON HICKS CONTRACTIONS

FERTILISATION

The process by which the man's sperm penetrates the woman's ovum in the Fallopian tube and creates a new human. Fertilisation can only occur if intercourse takes place up to 48 hours before or 24 hours after ovulation occurs. Family planning clinic staff teach women that sperm can live longer than 48 hours.

FETAL DEVELOPMENT

The growth of the baby during pregnancy. The brain, heart, lungs, kidneys and liver, the central nervous system and the digestive tract develop during the first three months. From then on, development is mainly in terms of the baby increasing in size.

FETAL SAC

➤ AMNIOTIC SAC

FETUS

The medical term for the baby from the fourth month of pregnancy to the time when he is born.

FIRST STAGE

The first part of labour when contractions cause the cervix or neck of the womb to open up to 10cm. May last from a few hours to a few days, but generally between 12 and 18 hours with a first baby.

FLUID RETENTION

The volume of your blood increases dramatically during pregnancy and fluid accumulates in your tissues. Your ankles, hands and face may become puffy. Always mention any swelling to your midwife as it can sometimes be a sign of pre-eclampsia.

➤ PRE-ECLAMPSIA; OEDEMA

FOLIC ACID

Vitamin that helps prevent spina bifida. You should take 400 micrograms a day from the time you start trying to get pregnant to three months after you become pregnant. Women who have already had a baby with this condition should take a higher dose. Your doctor will advise you on how much to take and when to begin.

FORCEPS

Forceps help your baby to be born if he is in an awkward position or you have become exhausted during the pushing part of labour. Curved stainless steel 'blades' are placed round the baby's head and the doctor pulls while you push.

FOREMILK

This is the first milk to come out of the breast when your baby feeds. It is thin and watery and quenches her thirst. The rich hindmilk comes after and satisfies her appetite.

FUNDUS

The top of the uterus which reaches your belly button by 20 weeks of pregnancy, your diaphragm by 36 weeks, and then drops down again as the baby engages in the pelvis. Contractions start at the fundus and radiate round to the cervix.

➤ ENGAGEMENT

GAS AND AIR

➤ ENTONOX

GENITAL HERPES

Painful ulcers (similar to cold sores) on the genital area. If the ulcers are 'active' or weepy at the end of pregnancy, it is safer for the baby to be born by caesarean to avoid the ulcers infecting his eyes and possibly causing blindness.

GERMAN MEASLES

Another name for rubella. If you catch it for the first time in early pregnancy, your baby's heart, brain and eyes may be affected. If caught later in pregnancy, the baby is less at risk although his hearing may be damaged.

GINGIVITIS

Medical term for inflammation of the gums. Common in pregnancy and can lead to tooth decay. Visit your dentist regularly – dental treatment is free until your baby is one year old.

GLUCOSE TOLERANCE TEST

A test for diabetes. After you have fasted for six hours, your blood sugar level is measured. You are given a glucose drink and then further blood tests are carried out. Your blood sugar level should rise initially, and then quickly return to normal.

GUTHRIE TEST

A test using a spot of your baby's blood taken from his heel when he is about four days old to detect a rare disease called phenylketonuria. The same blood sample is also used to test for thyroid and sugar disorders. If phenylketonuria is present a special diet is needed.

HAEMOGLOBIN

The iron-containing part of your blood that makes it red. Lack of haemoglobin causes

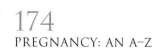

anaemia. Haemoglobin levels are tested at your booking visit, and at 28 and 36 weeks. It's normal for haemoglobin levels to drop slightly during pregnancy, as the volume of blood circulating rises. Anaemia can cause tiredness and breathlessness. Iron supplements can alleviate these symptoms.

HAEMORRHAGE

Haemorrhage means bleeding, and an antepartum haemorrhage is when you lose blood from the vagina during pregnancy – tell your GP or midwife immediately. A postpartum haemorrhage sometimes happens in the third stage of labour, or up to 10 days after birth if some of the placenta has been left in the womb. If bleeding is sudden and heavy call an ambulance.

➤ THIRD STAGE

HAEMORRHOIDS

These are varicose veins in the back passage. They are often extremely painful and may bleed profusely. Constipation makes them worse so eat plenty of cereal, wholemeal bread, fresh fruit and vegetables and drink plenty of fluids. Your doctor will be able to prescribe a suitable ointment to help shrink and soothe piles. Some women find that grated raw potato placed directly on the haemorrhoids is soothing.

HCG – HUMAN CHORIONIC GONADOTROPHIN

The hormone measured by pregnancy tests. At 18 weeks of pregnancy, the level of HCG in your blood can be used to estimate your risk of having a baby with Down's syndrome.

HIV

Human Immunodeficiency Virus transmitted through sexual intercourse. If you are HIV positive, talk to your midwife and obstetrician about combination drug treatment. It may be safer for you to give birth by caesarean, and not to breastfeed. Not all babies will inherit the HIV antibodies from their mother, and the right care during pregnancy can minimise the risks to the baby.

➤ AIDS

HOMOEOPATHY

Homoeopathic medicines stimulate the body to heal itself. Homoeopathy defines health as the harmonious interaction of mind, body and spirit. A qualified homoeopath can prescribe remedies for many disorders of pregnancy and the postnatal period. There is little research evidence for the effectiveness of homoeopathic remedies but much anecdotal evidence.

HORMONES

Chemical messengers such as oestrogen and adrenalin which bring about changes in the body. Progesterone is the hormone that sustains pregnancy. Oxytocin is the hormone that makes your womb contract in labour, and prolactin stimulates breast milk production.

HYDROTHERAPY

Exercising in water during pregnancy to keep fit, relieve aches and pains, and enjoy being weightless for an hour!

HYPNOTHERAPY

A hypnotherapist helps you achieve a state between waking and sleeping where you can deal with emotional problems and irrational fears. You can be taught to hypnotise yourself as a means of controlling pain during labour. Always consult someone properly qualified.

IMMUNE SYSTEM

Infections, such as chickenpox, cause your body to manufacture antibodies which prevent you from catching it again. The immune system is made up of all the antibodies which you have acquired either from having infections or as a result of being vaccinated.
➤ ANTIBODIES; IMMUNISATION; VACCINATION

IMMUNISATION

You should not have any immunisations during pregnancy. If possible, defer travelling to countries for which immunisations are required. If you are non-immune to rubella, you will be offered immunisation after the birth and should not become pregnant again for three months.
➤ VACCINATION

IMPLANTATION

This occurs when the cluster of cells that are the beginning of the new baby embed in the wall of the womb about seven days after fertilisation. You may find that you have a some 'spotting' at this time called an implantation bleed.

INCONTINENCE

Loss of control over bladder or bowels. Pushing for hours in the second stage of labour, or having a forceps or ventouse delivery, make you more prone to incontinence. Your physiotherapist should be able to help.
➤ SECOND STAGE

INVOLUTION

The process by which the womb shrinks after childbirth and returns to its pre-pregnant size and position. This takes about six weeks. The hormones involved in breastfeeding make involution more efficient.

ITCHING

Women who have a scar on their abdomen may find it becomes very itchy during pregnancy. You should always report any itching to your midwife or GP, especially if your entire body is involved, as it may be a sign of obstetric cholestasis.
➤ OBSTETRIC CHOLESTASIS

KEGEL EXERCISES

➤ PELVIC FLOOR EXERCISES

KETONES

Produced when the body breaks down fat, rather than burning sugar to meet its energy requirements. Your urine is tested for ketones during labour and you may be advised to have a glucose drip if they are present. Avoid this happening by eating regular snacks during early labour.

KICK CHART

One way of monitoring the well-being of the unborn baby using a chart for you to record movements of the baby. The usefulness of kick charts has not been established by research and some mothers find them anxiety-provoking.

LAMAZE METHOD

Method of preparation for childbirth devised by Fernand Lamaze in the 1950s. Involves learning detailed breathing patterns for coping with contractions. Most teachers incorporate some Lamaze-based teaching into their classes.

LEBOYER METHOD

The French obstetrician Frederic Leboyer felt that babies should be born into an environment similar to that of the womb in order to reduce psychological trauma. He therefore advocated dimming the lights at the moment of birth, and immersing the baby immediately in warm water.

LIGAMENTS

The ligaments supporting your back and pelvic joints soften during pregnancy, so that the pelvis will stretch to make more room for your baby. Softening can make the joints abnormally mobile. If overstretched, they become painful. They can also be more prone to injury and this can last up to six months after the baby is born.
➤ BACKACHE

LINEA NIGRA

Increased skin pigmentation during pregnancy may cause a dark line to appear down the middle of the abdomen. This fades after the baby is born.

LISTERIOSIS

An infection caught from eating unwashed fruit and vegetables, or soft cheeses made from unpasteurised milk. While the pregnant woman may have only a brief flu-like illness, the unborn baby may be seriously affected leading to death or premature birth.

LITHOTOMY POSITION

A position in which the woman lies on the delivery bed with her legs raised and held apart in stirrups to enable certain medical procedures such as a forceps delivery to be carried out. Often used when tears or cuts are stitched.

LOCHIA

The name given to the blood that you lose for two to three weeks after giving birth. To begin with, the loss is like a heavy period with bright red blood that may contain clots. Later, the flow decreases and becomes brownish in colour. It can continue for as long as six weeks.
➤ SEE PAGE 117

LOW BIRTHWEIGHT

A white baby who weighs under 2,500g is considered to be of low birthweight, but low birthweight for babies in other racial groups may be less than this. Low birthweight babies are vulnerable to infection, illness and breathing difficulties.

MASSAGE

Massage stimulates the body to release endorphins or natural pain-killing substances. Labouring women often appreciate firm rhythmical pressure applied to their lower back. Massage techniques can be learnt in antenatal classes.

MASTITIS

An infection of the breast. Breastfeeding women are often incorrectly diagnosed as having mastitis when their problem is a blocked milk duct causing localised inflammation. Antibiotics are appropriate for mastitis, but feeding the baby on the affected side is the solution for a blocked duct.

MECONIUM

The baby's first bowel movement is black, sticky and tar-like. Sometimes a baby opens her bowels in the womb during labour, turning the waters a muddy colour. Meconium staining of the waters may be a sign that the baby is distressed.

MEMBRANES

➤ AMNIOTIC SAC

MENSTRUAL CYCLE

The number of days from the start of one period to the start of the next – on average 28. Tell your midwife if your cycle is shorter or longer than the norm because this will affect her calculation of your expected date of delivery.

MIDWIFE

A specialist in normal pregnancy and birth. The word means 'with the wife'. Midwives care for women during pregnancy, deliver babies and give postnatal care and support.

MINERALS

Substances such as iron, calcium, magnesium and zinc which are found in a well-balanced diet. Your body needs minerals especially during pregnancy. Check that you are eating dark green leafy vegetables such as spinach, and plenty of wholemeal bread, unrefined cereals, dairy products and fish.

MOXIBUSTION

A technique used in traditional Chinese medicine for turning breech babies into a head-down position. A herb called 'moxa' is burned close to acupuncture points on the mother's feet. Success rates are reported to be as high as 90%.

MULTIGRAVIDA

This refers to a woman having a second or subsequent pregnancy. It may be shortened to multip.

NAUSEA

Feeling sick without vomiting is common in the first three months of pregnancy. Eat regular small snacks – ginger and peppermint are particularly comforting. Pethidine, used in labour for pain relief, may cause nausea. An injection of an anti-sickness drug should help and is usually given at the same time as pethidine.

NIPPLES

The key to preventing your nipples from becoming sore when breastfeeding is to ensure your baby is correctly latched on. Ask your midwife/breastfeeding counsellor for help. In labour, stimulating the nipples may make contractions more effective.

NOSEBLEEDS

It's not uncommon to have nosebleeds in pregnancy as a result of the increased volume of blood in your circulation which places extra pressure on the tiny vessels in your nose.

NUCHAL TRANSLUCENCY SCAN

A screening test carried out at 12 weeks of pregnancy using a high resolution ultrasound scanner to measure the fold of skin behind the baby's neck. The thickness of the fold correlates with the risk of Down's syndrome.

OBSTETRIC CHOLESTASIS

A serious complication of pregnancy involving the liver and bile duct. The mother experiences relentless itching over her whole body. Both she and the baby are at risk, and the pregnancy needs careful monitoring in a consultant unit.

OBSTETRICIAN

A doctor who is specially trained to care for women during pregnancy, labour and the early postnatal period. The obstetrician's expertise is best used in an emergency situation; the expert in normal childbearing is your midwife.

OCCIPITO-ANTERIOR (OA) POSITION

➤ ANTERIOR POSITION

OEDEMA

Medical term for swelling. Some swelling, especially of the ankles and feet, is common in pregnancy. Sudden swelling may sometimes be a sign of pre-eclampsia.
➤ FLUID RETENTION; PRE-ECLAMPSIA

OESTROGEN

In pregnancy, oestrogen causes the muscles of the uterus to grow bigger and stimulates the development of milk glands in the breasts. At the end of pregnancy, oestrogen levels increase and this is one factor that initiates labour.

OPERCULUM

➤ SHOW

ORGASM

The climax of sexual intercourse. Although the uterus contracts strongly when the woman reaches orgasm, the contractions melt away in a few moments and will not stimulate labour unless labour is about to start anyway.

OSTEOPATHY

A form of health care that depends on correcting the alignment of the bones of the body and ensuring that the muscles are free from tension. It is particularly useful during pregnancy when the muscular-skeletal system comes under unusual strain.

OVERDUE

Your baby is overdue when your pregnancy has passed 40 weeks. Going one week over your due date will not harm your baby. After 42 weeks, there is a case for inducing labour because the placenta may start to function less well.

OVULATION

The release of an egg once a month from the ovaries. Ovulation occurs 14 days before the start of menstruation, so if your menstrual cycle lasts 34 days, your best chance of becoming pregnant is to have intercourse 20 days from the first day of your last period.
➤ MENSTRUAL CYCLE

OXYTOCIN

The hormone that makes your womb contract during labour. It also causes milk to be squeezed out of the milk reservoirs in your breasts when your baby suckles.

PASSIVE IMMUNITY

The immunity a baby acquires from the antibodies passed to him by his mother during pregnancy and in breastfeeding. Colostrum is especially rich in antibodies which is why breastfeeding protects babies against infection.

PELVIC FLOOR EXERCISES

Exercises designed to strengthen the muscles of the pelvic floor. Your midwife, physiotherapist or antenatal teacher can show you how to do them. Practising regularly reduces your risk of incontinence and prolapse.
➤ PROLAPSE

PERINEUM

The tissue that extends from the back of your vagina to the back passage. It can be protected from tearing if you gently breathe the baby's

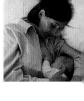

head out when you give birth rather than pushing forcibly. The definition of perineum as taught to medical students is the vulval area from the lower edge of the pubic symphysis backwards. This includes urethra and vaginal orifice.
➤ EPISIOTOMY

PESSARY

A vaginal suppository. Prostaglandin pessaries are used to induce labour when the cervix is not 'ripe' (ready for labour). They make the cervix soften and shorten and this will often stimulate contractions to start. Thrush, which is more common in pregnancy, is also treated by pessaries. It is normal for pessaries to melt at body temperature.

PETHIDINE

Synthetic form of morphine used for pain relief in labour. Given by injection into the thigh. May make you drowsy and sick; also passes to the baby and can make him more difficult to breastfeed. Some women find pethidine relaxing, others that it makes then feel out of control.

PHENYLKETONURIA

A condition affecting 1 in 10,000 babies. The baby cannot properly metabolise proteins, and the partially broken down by-products accumulate in the brain causing mental retardation. Can be detected using the Guthrie test and treated by diet so that the baby develops normally.

PICA

Craving for strange things to eat during pregnancy. Some women have a compulsion to eat coal or newspaper; others crave food they would not normally enjoy, or large quantities of food they normally eat only in small quantities, if they can bear to eat it at all.

PILES

➤ HAEMORRHOIDS

PLACENTA

The amazing organ that passes oxygen, food and antibodies from the mother to the baby in the womb. While it acts as a barrier to many harmful substances, it cannot stop drugs, nicotine and viruses from reaching the baby.

PLACENTA PRAEVIA

Condition requiring caesarean section when the placenta is situated close to the cervix, or lies across it. At the 20 weeks scan, many placentas look as if they are near the cervix, but 'move away' when the lower part of the uterus stretches later in pregnancy.

PRE-ECLAMPSIA

A disease of the placenta. Develops after 20 weeks and is more common with first babies and in women with a family history of pre-eclampsia. The mother has high blood pressure, protein in the urine, and sometimes, swelling.
➤ ECLAMPSIA

PREMATURE BIRTH

Birth occurring before 37 completed weeks of pregnancy. Premature babies may have difficulty breathing, maintaining their body temperature and sucking and often need the support of a special care baby unit. You'll find more information on pre-term babies and their care on pages 146 and 147.

PRESENTATION

The term midwives use to describe the part of the baby that is most deeply engaged in the

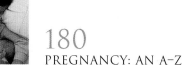

pelvis and which is likely to be born first. The most usual presentations are cephalic or vertex (head first) or breech (bottom first).

➤ ENGAGEMENT

PRE-TERM

Another word for 'premature'. Often used in the phrase 'pre-term rupture of membranes' which means that the mother's waters have broken before she has reached 37 weeks of pregnancy.

PRIMAGRAVIDA

This refers to a woman in her first pregnancy. It is sometimes shortened to primip.

PROGESTERONE

High levels of progesterone keep you pregnant, preventing the womb from pushing your baby out too soon. Progesterone also relaxes the muscles in your gut and urinary tract which can lead to indigestion, constipation and urinary infections.

PROLACTIN

Stimulates your breasts to make milk and dampens down production of the hormone that triggers the menstrual cycle. This is why breastfeeding can have a contraceptive effect, but this will be reduced if you introduce formula milk and when you wean your baby.

PROLAPSE

If the muscles of the pelvic floor are weak, they cannot support the bladder, vagina and womb. These organs then collapse or prolapse into each other, leading to infection and incontinence. Practising pelvic floor muscle exercises or 'kegels' helps prevent prolapse.

➤ SEE PAGE 37

PSYCHOPROPHYLAXIS

A method of preparing women for labour which attempts to break into the cycle of fear leading to tension leading to pain by helping women understand what happens during labour (so reducing fear) and acquire relaxation skills (so reducing tension) leading to a reduction in pain.

PTYALISM

Excessive production of saliva experienced by some women from as early as 8 weeks of pregnancy. No cures are known; spitting into a tissue prevents the stomach from becoming overloaded with subsequent sickness and loss of appetite.

PUDENDAL BLOCK

An anaesthetic injection given via the vagina or through the perineum to numb the nerves serving the lower part of the vagina, the perineum and the vulva. Sometimes used before a forceps delivery is carried out.

PUERPERAL PSYCHOSIS

Serious mental illness affecting 1 in 1,000 women. The woman breaks down within days of giving birth, suffering from hallucinations and insomnia, and losing touch with reality. She may harm herself or her baby. Admission to hospital, preferably to a mother and baby consultant, is necessary.

PUERPERIUM

The six weeks following the birth of a baby.

QUICKENING

Quickening is when you first feel your baby moving inside you. With a first baby, quickening happens at about 20 weeks of pregnancy. With a second or subsequent baby, you may feel the first movements as early as 14 weeks.

RASPBERRY LEAF

Herbal remedy taken either as tea or in tablet form from about 36 weeks of pregnancy to tone the muscle of the uterus in preparation for labour. It's especially useful after labour to help the womb regain its pre-pregnancy size quickly.

RELAXATION

Many women learn relaxation techniques for the first time at antenatal classes. Being able to relax during labour helps you stay in control, conserve energy, and maximise the oxygen supply to your baby.

RELAXIN

A hormone that, in animals, softens the pelvic ligaments and the cervix in readiness for labour. No one is sure if it plays a part in human pregnancy.

RETAINED PLACENTA

Usually the placenta is expelled soon after the baby is born. Occasionally this does not happen and it is retained in the uterus. A manual removal may need to be performed.

RHESUS FACTOR

People whose red blood cells carry the rhesus factor are rhesus positive and whose cells don't are rhesus negative. The blood of a rhesus negative mother may attack the cells of a rhesus positive baby and destroy them. So rhesus negative women have regular blood tests during pregnancy, and if necessary are given an injection after the birth which will protect subsequent babies.

RUBELLA

The medical term for German measles. If you catch the rubella virus during the first 16 weeks of pregnancy, your baby may develop heart, eye and hearing problems. Some women choose to terminate their pregnancy if infection is confirmed.

SACRUM

The lower part of your spine just above your tailbone. It is designed so that it can move backwards to make room for your baby to be born. To allow this to happen, you need to remain upright and mobile in labour.

SALIVA

Saliva tests are used to diagnose whether someone is a carrier of the cystic fibrosis gene. Genetic counselling is offered to couples who are both carriers because of the high risk of their babies having the disease.
➤ PTYALISM

SALMONELLA

A bacteria that causes food poisoning. It is found in raw meat and partly cooked eggs, so it's best to avoid home-made mayonnaise and any foods that have raw eggs in them while you are pregnant, and to wash your hands carefully after handling meat.

SCREENING

Blood tests and scans carried out in pregnancy to tell you what your risk is of having a baby with Down's syndrome or spina bifida. Screening tests can't guarantee that your baby is healthy (or say for certain that he is unhealthy). They are generally the first tests to be offered because they don't carry a miscarriage risk.

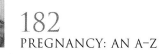

SECOND STAGE

The second stage of labour starts when the cervix is 10cm dilated and the pressure of your baby's head stimulates the nerves supplying your back passage, making you want to push. Second stage is completed when your baby is born.

SHIATSU

A Japanese form of healing that involves stretching exercises and placing pressure on the energy lines of the body, especially those in the abdomen. Properly qualified practitioners are registered with the Shiatsu Society.

SHIRODKAR SUTURE

A rarely used procedure which involves inserting a stitch round the cervix to prevent it from opening too early in pregnancy, causing the baby to be born prematurely. The stitch is inserted at 14 weeks and removed at 37 weeks.

SHOW

The name given to the mucous plug (or operculum) sealing the cervix during pregnancy, and protecting the baby against infection from the vagina. When the cervix opens, the plug comes away, sometimes with a little blood. It is an early sign of labour.

SPINA BIFIDA

A condition where the bones of the baby's spine have not closed properly around the spinal cord so that the nerves are damaged. People with spina bifida may be paralysed from the waist down, or they may have very few symptoms.

STILLBIRTH

A baby who shows no signs of life at birth is described as stillborn. Often, the baby is known to have died in the womb before labour starts, but sometimes a baby can be stillborn unexpectedly. The SANDS organisation helps people who have suffered this tragedy.

STITCHES

If your perineum tears during labour, or you have an episiotomy, you will probably have some stitches to repair the wound, which you need to keep clean and dry. Some women find that taking arnica tablets will help stitches and bruising heal. Practising pelvic floor muscle exercises helps by encouraging blood flow.
➤ EPISIOTOMY; PELVIC FLOOR EXERCISES; PERINEUM

STRETCH MARKS

Red lines where the skin has been stretched across your thighs and/or tummy during pregnancy. There's no evidence that using creams either prevents or improves them. After your baby is born, the marks will fade and become silvery and far less noticeable.

SYNTOCINON

A synthetic form of oxytocin, the hormone produced by the body to stimulate contractions. It is used in induction and acceleration of labour in the form of a drip. You'll find some more information on how labour is induced or accelerated on pages 94 and 95.

SYNTOMETRINE

Drug given by injection into your thigh as your baby's shoulders are being born, to speed the delivery of the placenta/afterbirth. It may reduce blood loss at the end of labour, but it can have side effects for both mother and baby.
➤ THIRD STAGE

TENS

Stands for transcutaneous electrical nerve stimulation. Used for pain relief in labour. Pulses of electricity channelled through four pads placed on your back override the pain signals produced by contractions of the uterus, and increase the body's natural pain relievers.

THALASSAEMIA

A serious blood disorder affecting people from Africa, Asia, the Middle East and the Mediterranean. Symptoms include severe pain and anaemia. Treatment is by repeated transfusions. If both mother and father are thalassaemia carriers, their baby will be at risk.

THIRD STAGE

The final part of labour, after your baby is born, when the placenta is delivered. Can be either 'physiological' with no drugs, or 'managed' with syntometrine.
➤ SYNTOMETRINE

THRUSH

Fungal infection that causes itching and white scabs in the mouth, vagina or on the nipples. Mothers sometimes pass it on to their babies during breastfeeding. Both mother and baby need treatment, and the mother should continue to breastfeed.

TOXAEMIA

➤ ECLAMPSIA

TOXOPLASMOSIS

Parasite infection endemic in the cat world. If you catch it for the first time in pregnancy, your baby's eyes and brain may be affected. To minimise your risk, don't handle cat litter, wash vegetables and fruit thoroughly, and don't eat undercooked meat.

TRANSITION

The bridge between the first and second stages of labour when your cervix is almost fully dilated and you start to feel the urge to push. Symptoms may include vomiting, shivering, aggressive behaviour and feelings of hopelessness.
➤ FIRST STAGE; SECOND STAGE

TRANSVERSE LIE

A midwifery term to describe a baby who is lying across his mother's womb so that neither his head nor his bottom is in her pelvis. These babies can only be born by caesarean section.

TRIAL OF LABOUR

If you have had a previous difficult delivery, or you have had problems during this pregnancy, you might choose a trial of labour to see if you can deliver your baby normally, while accepting that there is a strong possibility that labour will end in a caesarean.

TRIMESTER

A period of three months. Pregnancy is divided into three trimesters, first, middle and last.

TRIPLE TEST

➤ BART'S TEST

ULTRASOUND SCAN

An image of the internal organs of the body is produced on a screen by using the echoes of pulsed sound. Pregnancy scans can establish how many babies you are carrying, check the

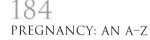

baby's growth and development and estimate your due date.

UMBILICAL CORD

The lifeline linking the baby to the placenta and hence to the mother. It contains three blood vessels: two arteries and one vein. Average length 50cm. May go on pulsating for some time after the baby is born. It is covered in a jelly-like substance (Wharton's jelly) which helps prevent it tangling.

UNSTABLE LIE

Term used by midwives to describe a baby whose position in the womb after 36 weeks of pregnancy keeps changing, rather than remaining head down or bottom down.

URINE TESTING

An important part of your pregnancy care. Protein in the urine may indicate that you have pre-eclampsia, or a urinary or vaginal infection. (However, it may also be due to contamination of the sample.)

UTERUS

The technical term for the womb. Composed of three layers: the inner layer which is shed monthly during menstruation; the middle or muscular layer, and the outer covering. The muscular layer grows enormously during pregnancy in preparation for labour.
➤ OESTROGEN

VACCINATION

A method of preventing serious diseases such as polio, diphtheria and tetanus by injecting into the body the organisms or an extract from the organisms that cause the disease in a modified form. The body responds by producing antibodies which prevent you from catching the disease.
➤ IMMUNISATION

VACUUM EXTRACTION

A way of helping the baby to be born if you are finding pushing too difficult. Involves placing a silicone plastic cup, called a ventouse cup, on the baby's head, sucking the air out, and then pulling on the cup to deliver the baby.
➤ SECOND STAGE

VAGINA

The passage between the cervix and the vulva which the baby travels down in order to be born. It is 10cm in length and its walls are very elastic so that they can stretch to accommodate the baby.
➤ VULVA

VARICOSE VEINS

Painful, distended veins in the legs or back passage. They are common in pregnancy because the weight of the baby obstructs blood flow to and from the legs. Wearing support tights or stockings can help with the symptoms. Try to avoid standing still for long periods of time.
➤ HAEMORRHOIDS

VENTOUSE

➤ VACUUM EXTRACTION

VERNIX

The greasy coating which covers the baby during the last months of pregnancy to help protect the baby's skin, and which means he is slippery and can travel more easily down the vagina during labour. Vernix is absorbed into the baby's body within a few hours of birth.

VITAMIN A

Important for good sight and for healing. Obtained from liver, fish, butter, egg yolk, cheese and many vegetables. Too much can be toxic, so you're safer to get your vitamin A from a healthy diet rather than from vitamin supplements.

VITAMIN K

Essential to make the blood clot. It is found in abundance in colostrum, and manufacturers add it to formula milk. Vitamin K used to be injected routinely into all new babies, but it is often given by mouth nowadays. Ask your midwife for details of what happens in your area.
➤ COLOSTRUM

VULVA

The outer part of the vagina, composed of thick layers of skin which form outer and inner lips or labia. The colour of the vulva changes from pink to purple during pregnancy.

WATERBIRTH

Women may choose to labour in water to ease the pain of contractions. Some go on to give birth underwater. The baby will not start to breathe until brought to the surface. Midwives often comment on how relaxed waterbirth babies appear to be.

WEIGHT GAIN

The mother's weight gain is not a good indicator of how well her baby is growing and many antenatal clinics no longer weigh women. There is little agreement on the optimum weight gain during pregnancy. The average is about 14kg, but it does vary a great deal. It is not a good idea to go on a diet during pregnancy.
Find more information on page 46.

WOMB

➤ UTERUS

X CHROMOSOME

The female sex chromosome. The egg which is released from the ovary each month contains an X chromosome, but male sperm contain either an X or a Y chromosome. If the egg is fertilised by a sperm carrying an X chromosome, the result will be a baby girl (XX).
➤ Y CHROMOSOME

X-RAYS

Still used occasionally during late pregnancy. If the mother has suffered an injury to her pelvis or spine, or has a bone disease, an x-ray is useful to assess whether she can deliver her baby normally, but no longer used in early pregnancy as it is considered unsafe for the developing baby. If you need dental treatment involving x-rays tell your dentist that you are pregnant.

Y CHROMOSOME

The male sex chromosome. If the egg is fertilised by a sperm carrying a Y chromosome, the result will be a baby boy (XY).
➤ X CHROMOSOME

ZINC

Important for the normal development of the baby in the womb, and to help strengthen the uterine muscles. The best sources of zinc are high-fibre foods such as bran cereals, hard cheese, meat and Brazil nuts.

ZYGOTE

The name given to the embryo in the very earliest stage of its development.

RESOURCES

Your midwife, family doctor or health visitor should be able to help you with any pregnancy-related queries you may have. In addition, here is a list of useful organisations to contact.

National Childbirth Trust
Alexandra House
Oldham Terrace
London W3 6NH
Tel: 020 8992 8637
Mon–Fri 9.30am–4.30pm

The NCT can give telephone help through the above Enquiries Line and put you in touch with your local NCT branch for antenatal classes, postnatal support groups and help from a breastfeeding counsellor. The NCT attempts to make its services, activities and membership fully accessible to everyone.

Health Information Service
Tel: 0800 665544 (England and Wales)
Tel: 0800 224488 (Scotland)
Tel: 0345 581929 (Northern Ireland)
A national network of NHS-funded helplines providing free, confidential information on keeping well, treatments, using health services, rights and complaints. Around 200 lines covering 26 centres, many of them open all day, every day.

STAYING WELL IN PREGNANCY
Sainsbury's/Wellbeing Helpline
Tel: 0114 242 4084
Mon–Fri 10am–4pm
For advice on what to eat during pregnancy and while breastfeeding.

Stopping smoking/Quitline
Tel: 0800 00 22 00, or try the

information on the internet at
www.healthnet.org.uk/quit/guide

Toxoplasmosis
Tel: 020 7593 1150
Up-to-date information, plus advice for women who may have been infected with toxoplasmosis during pregnancy.

The Anaphylaxis Campaign
Tel: 01252 542029
The British Allergy Foundation
Tel: 020 8303 8525
Both these organisations give support and guidance to people faced with allergy problems.

Aromatherapy
Putting you in touch with qualified practitioners:
The International Society of Professional Aromatherapists
Tel: 01455 637987
The Register of Qualified Aromatherapists
Tel: 01245 227957

Acupuncture
The British Acupuncture Council
Park House, 206–208 Latimer Road
London W10 6RE
Tel: 020 8735 0400

Homoeopathy
The British Homoeopathic Association
27A Devonshire Street
London W1N 1RJ
Tel: 020 7935 2163

Back care
General Osteopathic Council
Tel: 020 7357 6655
A recorded message will give you an option to select for the Osteopathic Information Service – for further information about osteopathy and details of osteopaths in your area.

Action on Pre-eclampsia (APEC)
31–33 College Road
Harrow
Middlesex
HA1 1EJ
Tel: 020 8427 4217

PLANNING THE BIRTH
Contacting an independent midwife
Independent Midwives Association
The Wessex Maternity Centre
Mansbridge Road
West End
Southampton
SO18 3HW
Enclose an A5 stamped, addressed envelope and you will be sent a register of all the independent midwives in the UK.

Finding a doula (birth companion)
Birth and Bonding International
60 Nottingham Road
Belper
DE56 1JH
Tel: 01773 826055
Write to them for a list of doulas.

Hiring a birthing pool
Aqua Birth Pool Hire
Tel: 01202 518152

Splashdown Water Birth Services
Tel: 020 8422 9308

Active Birth Centre
25 Bickerton Road
London N19 5JT
Tel: 020 7482 5554
Mon–Fri 9.30am–5.30pm
Sat 10am–4pm
Pre- and postnatal yoga classes,
preparation for birth and waterbirth
pool hire.

Caesarean Support Network
55 Cooil Drive
Douglas
Isle of Man
IM2 2HF
Tel: 01624 661269
Every day 6pm–10pm

National Childbirth Trust (see
above) also runs support groups for
women who have had a caesarean.

Birth Crisis Network
Tel: 020 7485 4725
or 01865 300266
or 0141 946 7537
Telephone help for women who felt
disempowered in childbirth and
want to talk about it.

EXPECTING MORE THAN
ONE BABY?
Twins and Multiple Births
Association (TAMBA)
Harnott House
309 Chester Road
Little Sutton
Ellesmere Port
CH66 1QQ
Tel: 0151 348 0020
Helpline: 01732 868000
Mon–Fri 7pm–11pm
Sat–Sun 10am–11pm
Information and support for parents
who are expecting (or who have)
twins, triplets, or more. TAMBA
runs local twins clubs and publishes
a newsletter too.

Multiple Births Foundation
020 8383 3519
Telephone counselling.

MATERNITY RIGHTS AT
WORK
Parents At Work
45 Beech Street
London EC2Y 8AD
Tel: 020 7628 3565
For advice and information on
childcare and employment issues
relating to pregnancy and working
parents. An answering machine
takes your call 24-hours a day. It
gives out another number for
personal attention, or you can
simply leave your address for an
information pack.

The Maternity Alliance
Tel: 020 7588 8582
An excellent source of information
and support on the rights for
women at work before and after
childbirth.

Daycare Trust
Shoreditch Town Hall Annexe
380 Old Street
London EC1V 9LT
Tel: 020 7739 2866
National childcare charity
campaigning to improve conditions
for the working parent.

National Childminding Association
(NCMA)
8 Masons Hill
Bromley
Kent BR2 9EY
Tel: 020 8466 0220
Mon–Tue 2.00-4.00pm
Thurs 1.00-3.00pm

PREMATURE BABIES
Bliss (Baby Life Support Systems)
2nd Floor
87–89 Albert Embankment
London SE1 7TP
Tel: 020 7820 9471

BABY LOSS
Antenatal Results and Choices
(ARC)
73–75 Charlotte Street
London W1P 1LB
Tel: 020 7631 0285

The Miscarriage Association
Clayton Hospital
Northgate
Wakefield
West Yorkshire
WF1 3JS
Tel: 01924 200799
Mon–Fri 9am–4pm

Stillbirth and Neonatal Death
Society (SANDS)
28 Portland Place
London W1N 4DE
Tel: 020 7436 5881
Mon–Fri 10am –5pm
Information and support groups.

Foundation for the Study of Infant
Deaths (FSID)
24-hour helpline:
Tel: 020 7235 1721

'SPECIAL NEEDS' BABIES
Birth Defects Foundation
Martindale
Hawksgreen
Cannock
Staffordshire
WS11 2XN
Tel: 01543 468400
Mon–Fri 9.30am–3pm
enquiries@birthdefects.co.uk
www.birthdefects.co.uk
Support and information for
families.

Association for Spina Bifida and
Hydrocephalus
ASBAH House
42 Park Road
Peterborough
PE1 2UQ
Tel: 01733 555988

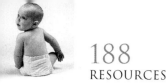

Cleft Lip and Palate Association
(CLAPA)
235–237 Finchley Road
London NW3 6LS
Tel: 020 7431 0033

Down's Syndrome Association
155 Mitcham Road
London SW17 9PG
Tel: 020 8682 4001
For children and their carers.

Contact-a-Family
Helping families of children with
'special needs'
Tel: 020 7383 3555

Disabled Parents Network
PO Box 5876
Towcester
NN12 7ZN
Supporting pregnancy & parenthood
for people with disabilities.

REACH – for hand/arm deficiency
Tel: 01933 274126

SCOPE
6 Market Road
London N7 9PW
Tel: 020 7619 7100
Tel: 0808 800 3333
Mon–Fri 9am–9pm
Sat–Sun 2pm–6pm
Help for children with cerebral
palsy and their carers.

Sickle Cell Society
54 Station Road
Harlesden
London NW10 4UA
Tel: 020 8961 7795
or 020 8961 4006
A national charity for sickle cell
sufferers.

NEED A FRIEND?
The National Childbirth Trust (see
above) runs local postnatal groups in
all areas where new parents can get
to know each other.

MAMA (Meet-a-Mum Association)
Tel: 020 8768 0123
Mon–Fri 7pm–10pm
MAMA is a nationwide group that
puts mums into contact with other
mums in their region. They also
hold study days.

Association for Post-Natal Illness
(APNI)
25 Jerdan Place
Fulham
London SW6 1BE
Tel: 020 7386 0868

Home-Start
2 Salisbury Road
Leicester
LE1 7QR
Tel: 0116 233 9955
Trained volunteers nationwide will
come to your home if you've just
had a baby and are under stress.

Positively Women
347–349 City Road
London EC1V 1LR
Tel: 020 7713 0222
Support for women with HIV and
AIDS and their families.

BREASTFEEDING
The National Childbirth Trust (see
above) can put you in touch with a
local NCT Breastfeeding Counsellor.
You don't need to join the NCT to
get this help.

La Leche League (Great Britain)
BM3424
London WC1N 3XX
Tel: 020 7242 1278
Breastfeeding help over the
telephone and a list of local level
support groups.

Association of Breastfeeding
Mothers (ABM)
Tel: 020 7813 1481
9am–5pm
Telephone support for breastfeeding.

WEBSITES
As more and more information is
becoming available online, people
who have access to the world-wide
web can search out answers they
need. A search engine such as Yahoo
is somewhere to start. Just key in:
http://dir.yahoo.com/health/reproduc
tive_health/pregnancy_and_birth for
a long list of organisations that
could be of interest. Also try:

www.nct-online.org
National Childbirth Trust (see above).

www.nctms.co.uk
NCT Maternity Sales – bras, birth
accessories, books, clothes and
products for new babies.

www.activebirthcentre.com
Active Birth Centre – birth
preparation classes, support and
practical advice; big supplier of
birthing pools.

www.babyworld.co.uk
New and expectant parents will enjoy
this interactive online magazine.

www.babycentre.co.uk
Another online organisation aimed
at new parents.

www.babydirectory.com
A series of locally based printed
guides containing a wide variety of
information for new parents, which
are also accessible online.

www.dss.gov.uk/ba/maternity
Department of Social Security. Click
on 'Benefits Agency' for straight
information about maternity pay.

www.womens-health.co.uk
For up-to-date health information.

www.medscape.com
You can find the latest medical
research here on one site.

INDEX

abdominal pain 60
abdominal transducers 97
abruptio placenta 66
accelerating labour 95
active births 166
acupuncture 39
AFP tests 166
afterbirth *see* placenta
afterpains 166
AIDS (Acquired Immune
    Deficiency Syndrome) 166
air travel 23, 45, 73
alcohol consumption 10, 13,
    20
allergies 166
amniocentesis 31–2, 62, 166
amniofiltration 167
amniotic fluid 167
amniotic sac 167
anaemia 59, 174
analgesia *see* pain relief
    (analgesia)
'anomaly' scans 45
antenatal care 15, 24–5, 26,
    55, 62
antenatal classes 15, 42–5,
    168
    time off work for 55
antenatal tests 15, 30–3, 62,
    166–7
    diagnostic 30, 31–2
    see also blood tests
anterior (occiput-anterior)
    position 167
antibiotics 167
antibodies 167
anxiety 167
Apgar scores (babies) 48,
    155, 167
areola 168
arnica tablets 118, 166, 182
aromatherapy 21, 168
artificial respiration, for
    newborn babies 143

baby blues 121
baby carriers 125
baby's heartbeat, monitoring
    during labour 96–7
back strain/backache 46–7,
    62, 168
    during labour 86, 87
Bart's test 168
benefits (state) 45, 54, 56
birth of the baby 85, 102–11
    assisted deliveries 106–7,
        132
        forceps 50, 95, 106,
            107, 170, 173, 176,
            180
        ventouse 50, 95, 106,
            107, 184
    birth stories 148–65
    breastfeeding after 132
    positions for 76
    twins or more 63, 162–3
    your body after the birth
        116–19
    see also caesarean section
Birth and Bonding
    International 52–3
birth coaches (doulas) 52–3,
    170
birth plans 50–1, 73, 99
birthing pools *see* waterbirths
bleeding
    decidual 13
    in early pregnancy 14–15,
        65
    implantation 175
    in later pregnancy 66
    problems with 64–6
bleeding gums 41
blood pressure 168
blood tests 26, 31, 45, 62,
    181
    AFP 166
    Bart's test 168
    cordocentesis 170
    Guthrie test 173, 179

on newborn babies 115
    and pre-eclampsia 66
    and the rhesus factor 67
bonding 168
booking visit 26–7
bottle-feeding 129–31,
    138–41
    advantages of 129
    and baby's bowel motions
        114–15
    by other people 140–1
    choosing formula milk
        130–1
    equipment for 130, 131,
        138
    positions 138–9
    and soya-based milk 131
    sterilising feeding
        equipment 141
bowel motions, newborn
    babies 114–15
bras for breastfeeding 129
Braxton Hicks contractions
    70, 168, 172
breaking waters *see* waters
    breaking
breastfeeding 56, 126,
    128–9, 132–7, 168
    advantages of 127, 128,
        129, 166
    after the birth 132
    after a caesarean birth
        136–7, 157
    'after pains' 117
    baby-led 135–6
    and baby's bowel
        motions/wet nappies
        114, 115
    benefits for mothers 128,
        129
    colostrum 169, 178, 185
    combining with bottle-
        feeding 128, 131
    contraceptive effect of
        180

engorgement 171
equipment for 129, 132
expressing milk 147
foremilk 173
frequency of feeds 136
getting started 132–5
hindmilk 173
and involution 175
jaundiced babies 144
and mastitis 176
pain during 135, 177
premature babies 146,
    147
sleepy newborn babies
    143
and thrush 183
twins or more 63
breasts 40, 116–17, 176
    nipples 135, 168, 177
breathing
    during labour 74, 90,
        102, 103
    exercises 168
breathing difficulties (babies)
    142–3, 146
breathlessness (during
    pregnancy) 60, 70, 168
breech presentation 63,
    154–5, 177, 180
brow presentation 168

caesarean section 99, 108–9
    and the birth plan 50
    birth stories 154–7
    breastfeeding after 136–7,
        157
    elective 108, 109, 157
    emergency 108, 109,
        154–5, 156–7, 158
    and multiple births 63,
        100
    and placenta praevia 179
    and transverse lie 183
    vaginal birth after 158–9
    your body after 118–19

caffeine 21
cannabis 21
car safety 23
car seats 57, 58, 73, 79
carpal tunnel syndrome 61, 169
cephalic position 169
cerebral palsy 169
cervical erosion 65
cervical incompetence 169
cervical mucus 169
cervix 169
chlamydia 169
chlamydia psittaci 13
chloasma 169
chorionic villus sampling see CVS
clothes (baby) 57, 73
Community Health Council 24, 27
community-based care 25
complementary therapies 80, 158, 181
conception 12–15
congenital problems 30, 146, 147
constipation 40, 60, 170
contractions 84–5, 86, 87, 88, 170
    afterpains 166
    Braxton Hicks 70, 168, 172
    and breathing rhythm 90
    giving birth 102
cordocentesis 170
cot death 127
counselling 147
CPD (cephalo-pelvic disproportion) 169
cramp in legs 60, 170
CT scans 156
CVS (chorionic villus sampling) 30, 31, 62, 169
cystic fibrosis, tests for 181
cystitis 170

deafness, early diagnosis and treatment of 115
decidual bleeding 13
deep transverse arrest 170
dental treatment 15, 41, 185
diabetes 13, 94, 101, 170
    glucose test for 173
    and hypoglycaemia 145
    pregnancy-related 67, 170

diamorphine 93
diet 16–17
disabled women 100–1
discomforts in pregnancy 40–1, 59–61, 70, 73, 83–4
dizziness 40–1
domino scheme 170
doulas (birth coaches) 52–3, 170
Down's syndrome 170–1
    antenatal tests for 30, 31–2, 166, 169, 174, 181
drugs
    anti-malaria 23
    medication 10, 13, 20
    taking care with 20–1

'ear trumpet' (fetal stethoscope) 96
eclampsia 171
ectopic pregnancies 64, 65, 171
ECV (external cephalic version) 172
EDD (estimated date of delivery) 14, 73, 171
effleurage 171
embryo 171
emotions
    after the birth 103–4, 120–1, 124
    after a miscarriage 15, 64
    during labour 88, 89
    on giving birth prematurely 146–7
    mothers of babies with congenital problems 147
    in pregnancy 14, 41, 70, 82
endometrium 171
enema 171
engagement (of the baby's head) 171
engorgement 171
Entonox (gas and air) 48, 92–3, 171–2
    experiences of using 150–1, 152–3, 164–5
    and waterbirths 48, 149
epidurals 51, 92, 93, 106, 172
    and birth positions 76
    and caesarean sections 108, 109, 118
    'mobilising' 93

epilepsy 13
episiotomies 51, 172
    stitches after 117, 182
    and waterbirths 48
equipment
    for home births 79
    for the new baby 57–8
exercises
    antenatal 34–7
    keeping fit in pregnancy 15, 22–3
    pelvic tilting 47
    postnatal 122–3
    tummy strengtheners 37, 122
    see also pelvic floor exercises

fallopian tubes 172
family relationships, changing 69
feeding see bottle-feeding; breastfeeding
feelings see emotions
fertilisation 172
fetal (amniotic) sac 167
fetal blood sampling 97
fetal development 172
    first trimester 10, 12, 13
    second trimester 42
    third trimester 70
fluid retention 172–3
folic acid
    food rich in 17
    supplements 10, 13, 45, 173
food
    changing tastes in 38, 41
    eating after the birth 125
    eating well 16–17
    and pregnancy sickness 38, 39
food poisoning 18–19, 181
forceps deliveries 50, 95, 106, 107, 170, 173, 176, 180
fundus 173

gas and air see Entonox (gas and air)
genetic conditions 30, 166
genital herpes 94, 173
German measles see rubella
gestation, estimating 14
gestational diabetes 67, 170
gingivitis 173
glucose tolerance test 173

GPs (general practitioners) 20, 24, 26, 27, 115
gums, bleeding 41
Guthrie test 173, 179

haemoglobin 173–4
haemorrhage 174
HCG (human chorionic gonadotrophin) 12, 38, 174
headaches 40
health visitors 137
heartburn 39, 59, 62, 84
helplines 64, 147
high blood pressure 13, 66, 94
    see also pre-eclampsia
HIV (Human Immuno-deficiency Virus) 174
holidays 15, 23
home births 25, 73, 79, 86, 172
    advantages and disadvantages of 27
    birth stories 148–51, 158–9, 164–5
    waterbirths 49, 79, 148–9, 158–9
homoeopathy 174
hormones 174
hospital care 24, 25, 73, 90
    advantages and disadvantages of 27
    and baby blues 121
    birth stories 152–7, 160–3
    induced labour 80–1, 94–5
    leaving hospital with the new baby 124
    packing for 73, 78–9
    Special Care Baby Unit (SCBU) 63, 143, 146
    and waterbirths 48–9, 162–3
    when to go to hospital 87
    see also caesarean section
hydrotherapy 174
hypnotherapy 174
hypoglycaemia, and newborn babies 145

immune system 175
immunisations (vaccinations) 15, 23, 175, 184
implantation 175
incontinence 61, 175

inducing labour 80–1, 94–5
    birth story 160–1
infections 13
insomnia 61, 70
Internet 50
involution 116, 175
itching 60, 175, 177

jaundiced babies 144–5

kegel exercises *see* pelvic floor
    exercises
ketones 175
kick chart 175

labour 82–111
    accelerating 95
    and birth plans 50, 51
    clinical signs of 86–7
    deep transverse arrest 170
    encouraging labour to
        start 80
    experiences of 85
    false 172
    first stage 85, 86–9, 172
    induction 80–1, 94–5
    internal examinations
        during 89
    keeping moving 77
    latent phase of 98
    long labours 98–9
    making noises during 77,
        88
    and meconium-stained
        waters 99
    monitoring 96–7, 100,
        101
    old wives' tales about 82
    packing for 73, 78–9
    positions for 50, 51,
        74–6, 91, 103, 168
    positive thinking about
        77
    problematic 100–1
    quick labours 99
    relaxation during 74, 98
    second stage *see* birth of
        the baby
    skills for 74–7
    third stage 85, 110–11,
        183
    transition 89, 183
    trial of 183
    and waterbirths 48
    see also contractions;
        inducing labour; pain
        relief

labour companions/partners
    45, 52–3, 74, 75, 77
    at antenatal classes 44
    and the birth 102, 103
    and the birth plan 50, 51
    and disabled women 101
    and massage 76–7, 91
Lazame method 175
Leboyer method 175–6
leg cramps 60, 170
ligaments 176
linea nigra 176
listeria 18, 19, 176
lithotomy position 176
LMP (last monthly period)
    12, 13, 14, 80
lochia (vaginal loss) 116,
    117, 176

malaria 15, 23
massage 76–7, 91, 171, 176
mastitis 176
maternity allowance (MA)
    45, 54, 56
maternity leave 45, 54–5, 56
meconium, passed by
    newborn babies 114, 142,
    176
meconium-stained waters 99,
    176
medication, in the first
    trimester 10, 13
membranes (amniotic sac)
    176
menstrual cycle 177
Meptid 93
midwives 177
    and antenatal care 24, 25
    appointment with (at
        17–20 weeks) 45
    and the birth
        asking for assistance
            88
        delivery of the
            placenta 110
        waters breaking 87
        when to call 87
    booking visit 26–7
    daily checks after the
        birth 116
    and early pregnancy 14,
        15
    and help with
        breastfeeding 135, 137
    and home births 79, 158
    home care and newborn
        babies 112, 126

and information about
        assisted deliveries 106
    and labour partners 52
    and long labours 98–9
    monitoring labour 96–7
    selective visiting by 126
    and waterbirths 49
minerals 177
miscarriages 14–15, 20, 21,
    64
    and cervical incompetence
        169
    and CVS (chorionic villus
        sampling) 30
    following amniocentesis
        32
    'inevitable' 65
    and pregnancy sickness
        38
    'threatened' 65
mole pregnancies 64
morning sickness 38–9
mothers (of pregnant women)
    changing relationships
        with 69
    as labour partners 52
moxibustion 177

nappies 58, 114–15
NCT (National Childbirth
    Trust)
    breastfeeding counsellors
        137
    Special Experience
        Register 147
neonatal infection, and
    waterbirths 48
Neonatal Intensive Care Unit
    (NICU) 146
newborn babies 112–47
    Apgar scores 48, 155,
        167
    bottle-feeding 129–31,
        138–41
    breastfeeding 128–9,
        132–7
    breathing difficulties
        142–3
    early days at home 124–7
    equipment for 57–8
    health checks on 112,
        115
    holding close 105, 124,
        125
    and hypoglycaemia 145
    jaundiced 144–5
    low birthweight 176

nappies and bowel
        motions 58, 114–15
    premature 63, 145, 146,
        179
    reducing the risk of cot
        death 127
    sleeping 58, 127
    umbilical cord 110,
        112–14
NICU (Neonatal Intensive
    Care Unit) 146
nipples 135, 168, 177
nosebleeds 41, 177
notes, abbreviations on 29,
    33
Nuchal Translucency Test 31,
    62

obstetric cholestasis 177
obstetricians 177
oedema 178
oestrogen 178
operculum (show) 86, 182
orgasm 178
osteopathy 178
overdue babies 80–1, 94, 178
overweight 46
ovulation 178
oxygen, newborn babies short
    of 142–3
oxytocin 80, 117, 174, 178,
    182

pain relief (analgesia) 167
    after the birth 118
    after a caesarean 109
    and the birth plan 50, 51
    epidurals 51, 76, 92, 93,
        106
    helping yourself 90–1
    and induced labour
        160–1
    massage for 76–7, 91
    pethidine 93, 179
    and psychoprophylaxis
        180
    pudendal block 180
    TENS machines 73, 92,
        148, 152, 183
    and waterbirths 48
    see also Entonox (gas and
        air)
paracetamol 13, 20, 118
parasites 18
partners
    at antenatal classes 44
    changing relationships

with 68–9
and feelings after the
birth 120, 121
passive immunity 178
peanut allergies 19
pelvic floor exercises 37, 60,
61, 118, 122, 175, 178,
180, 182
pelvic tilting 47
perineum 118, 178–9
pessaries 179
prostaglandin 80–1, 94,
179
pethidine 93, 179
phenylketonuria 173, 179
pica 179
piles (haemorrhoids) 60, 174
placenta 18, 110–11, 142,
144, 179
abruption 66
delivery 50, 110, 182
low-lying (praevia) 66
and premature babies 146
retained 181
wound left by the 116
placenta praevia 179
postnatal exercises 122–3
posture 46–7
prams 57–8
pre-eclampsia 46, 61, 66–7,
168, 171, 173, 179
and induction 94
and premature babies 146
pregnancy-related diabetes
67
premature (pre-term) births
145, 146, 179
twins or more 63
presentation 179–80
primagravida 180
progesterone 38, 174, 180
prolactin 116, 174, 180
prolapse 180
protein foods 17
psychoprophylaxis 180
ptyalism 180
pudendal block 180
puerperal psychosis 180
puerperium 180
pushchairs 57–8

quickening 180–1

raspberry leaf 181
relaxation during labour 74,
98, 180, 181
relaxin 22, 181

retinol vitamin A 19
rhesus factor 67, 146, 181
rubella (German measles) 13,
18, 167, 173, 175, 181
runny nose 41

sacrum 181
safety 10, 18, 34, 55–6
saliva tests 181
salmonella poisoning 19, 181
scans see ultrasound scans
screening tests 30, 181
and blood sugar levels 67
Nuchal Translucency scan
31, 177
and twins or more 62
see also blood tests;
ultrasound scans
second pregnancies 69
second-hand equipment 57
sexual intercourse 65, 68, 80,
178
shared care 25
shiatsu 182
shirodkar suture 182
show (operculum) 86, 182
sickness in pregnancy 38–9
skin itching 60
skin pigmentation 42, 169,
176
sleeping
breastfeeding sleepy
babies 143
and newborn babies 58,
127
smoking 10, 13, 21, 127
sonicard (portable doppler)
96, 97
Special Care Baby Unit
(SCBU) 63, 143, 146
spina bifida 182
antenatal tests for 30, 31,
32, 166, 181
sports 10, 22
stillbirths 64, 182
stitches 107, 117, 182
stress incontinence 61, 175
stretch marks 42, 182
stuffy nose 41
swimming 22
swollen feet/ankles 61, 66,
70
symptoms of pregnancy
12–13
syntocinon drip 81, 94, 95,
182
syntometrine 182

talking over anxieties 41
talking to professionals 28–9
abbreviations on notes 29,
33
asking questions 26–7, 29
TAMBA (Twins and Multiple
Births Association) 62
team midwifery care 25, 27
TENS machines 73, 92, 148,
152, 183
tests
pregnancy tests 12, 13–14
urine 84, 126
see also antenatal tests;
blood tests; screening
tests
thalassaemia 183
thrush 41, 183
tiredness 10, 12, 40
toxaemia (eclampsia) 171
toxic substances 13
toxoplasmosis 18, 19, 183
toys for newborn babies 58
transverse lie 183
trial of labour 183
triple test (Bart's test) 168
twins and more 57, 62–3,
100
birth stories 162–3

ultrasound scans 32, 183–4
'anomaly' 45
and baby's rate of growth
94
CT 156
estimating gestation 14,
15, 32, 80
and twins or more 62
umbilical cord 110, 112–14,
184
unstable lie 184
urination 40
urine tests 26, 184
uterus 184
changes after the birth
116

vaccinations (immunisations)
15, 23, 175, 184
vacuum extraction 184
vagina 184
varicose veins 59, 62, 184
piles 60, 174
VBAC (vaginal birth after
caesarean) 158–9
ventouse deliveries 50, 95,
106, 107, 184

vernix 184
viruses 18
visitors, and newborn babies
125
vitamin A 19, 185
vitamin B$_6$ 39
vitamin D 17
vitamin K 51, 185
vulva 185

water, pain relief using 90–1
waterbirths 185
birth stories 148–9,
158–9, 162–3
birthing pools 45, 48–9,
75, 79
delivery of the baby 48
at home 49, 79, 148–9,
158–9
in hospital 48–9, 162–3
and labour positions 76
and pain relief 48
twin births 162–3
waters breaking 87, 94
inducing labour by 81,
94, 95
weight gain
of the baby 70
during pregnancy 46–7,
185
weights, working out with
34
winding 140
work
conditions unsuitable for
pregnant women 13
dismissal or redundancy
56
health and safety at 10,
55–6
and maternity leave 45,
54–5, 56
returning to 55, 56, 131
and Statutory Maternity
Pay (SMP) 54
taking time off 55, 62
telling employers about
the pregnancy 15

X chromosome 185
x-rays 185

Y chromosome 185

zinc 185
zygote 185